AD... ...d its Many Associated Problems

ADHD and Its Many Associated Problems

CHRISTOPHER GILLBERG

OXFORD
UNIVERSITY PRESS

OXFORD
UNIVERSITY PRESS

Oxford University Press is a department of the University of Oxford.
It furthers the University's objective of excellence in research, scholarship,
and education by publishing worldwide.

Oxford   New York
Auckland   Cape Town   Dar es Salaam   Hong Kong   Karachi
Kuala Lumpur   Madrid   Melbourne   Mexico City   Nairobi
New Delhi   Shanghai   Taipei   Toronto

With offices in
Argentina   Austria   Brazil   Chile   Czech Republic   France   Greece
Guatemala   Hungary   Italy   Japan   Poland   Portugal   Singapore
South Korea   Switzerland   Thailand   Turkey   Ukraine   Vietnam

Oxford is a registered trademark of Oxford University Press
in the UK and certain other countries.

Published in the United States of America by
Oxford University Press
198 Madison Avenue, New York, NY 10016

Library of Congress Cataloging-in-Publication Data
Gillberg, Christopher, 1950- author.
ADHD and its many associated problems / Christopher Gillberg.
   p. ; cm.
Includes bibliographical references.
ISBN 978–0–19–993790–5 (alk. paper)
I. Title.
[DNLM: 1. Attention Deficit Disorder with Hyperactivity.   2. Movement Disorders.
3. Sensation Disorders. WS 350.8.A8]
RC394.A85
616.85′89—dc23
2013030336

The science of medicine is a rapidly changing field. As new research and clinical experience broaden
our knowledge, changes in treatment and drug therapy occur. The author and publisher of this work
have checked with sources believed to be reliable in their efforts to provide information that is accurate
and complete, and in accordance with the standards accepted at the time of publication. However, in
light of the possibility of human error or changes in the practice of medicine, neither the author, nor
the publisher, nor any other party who has been involved in the preparation or publication of this work
warrants that the information contained herein is in every respect accurate or complete. Readers are
encouraged to confirm the information contained herein with other reliable sources, and are strongly
advised to check the product information sheet provided by the pharmaceutical company for each
drug they plan to administer.

9 8 7 6 5 4 3 2
Printed in the United States of America
on acid-free paper

CONTENTS

ADHD (attention-deficit/hyperactivity disorder) and its many associated problems (including developmental coordination disorder [DCD], oppositional defiant disorder [ODD], autism spectrum disorders [ASD], tic disorders, language disorder [LD], intellectual developmental disorder [IDD], reading and writing disorder, depression and anxiety disorders, to mention but the most common) are very common. Everyone meets children (and adults for that matter) with ADHD, DAMP (deficits in attention, motor control, and perception, also referred to as "ADHD with DCD"), or ESSENCE (Early Symptomatic Syndromes Eliciting Neurodevelopmental Clinical Examinations, a category that encompasses ADHD and all its early-onset associated problems) everyday. Everyone, at first, is more or less perplexed and will need an approach that rests on a humanistic foundation. This applies to an even greater degree to those who meet affected people in their professional lives. When "experts"—as still often happens—choose to bundle these types of diagnoses together indiscriminately and without any attempt at differential diagnosis, it shows that they do not take the issue seriously enough and that they—often because of ignorance—refuse or fail to deal with it. It is only with systematic knowledge that we can help children with special needs (and adults; children *do* grow up and problems often remain) in a long-term perspective, in a good way as fellow human beings, both in and out of school, in and out of the workplace, and within the health care system.

In this book, I shall attempt to summarize the information that we have about these children (and adolescents, and adults) with ADHD and its many associated neuropsychiatric problems (ESSENCE). As with all disabilities the impairment is relative and, to a considerable extent, determined by the person's environment. To be treated with understanding, respect, and insight is a fundamental condition for being able to feel a sense of belonging in society.

ADHD, DAMP, and ESSENCE are umbrella terms covering symptoms of variant/unusual/abnormal development associated with a number of important functions/dysfunctions in the brain. Many times, the symptoms are perceived as "normal" by the individual himself herself, but other people will usually consider him or her as being "different." Attentional functions are crucial for children to develop at an equal rate to their peers. To fit in at school or in other social situations is an important part of maturing. Being seen as "different" and not being met with understanding and appropriate expectations and demands creates a feeling of inadequacy. Knowing where to draw the line between different neuropsychiatric disabilities/ESSENCE, and where they overlap, is an important part of understanding how—in an optimal manner—one should face and interact with (and sometimes "treat") these children, and support them and their families.

For almost 40 years, my associates and I have been doing clinical work and research relating to children (and, for almost 20 years, adults) with early symptomatic neuropsychiatric disabilities/ESSENCE. Through a long series of scientific projects, papers, and books we have tried to spread information about ADHD and DAMP, ASD and learning disabilities, Tourette syndrome and DCD, eating disorders and psychosis, and, more recently, the other disorders subsumed under the ESSENCE acronym. This book summarizes the available information about these disorders in what I hope is an accessible manner and what is needed to face, support, and help children with these difficulties.

The frontiers of science are constantly being pushed forward. It is of crucial importance that scientific findings within the field reach both the relevant professionals and the general public. Approaching those who need support in an appropriate manner can be done only on the basis of solid information on the subject.

In this book, I shall attempt to convert scientific findings into a text that gives insight to specialists in child development, generalists, psychiatrists, clinical psychologists, and indeed to everyone touched by ADHD, DAMP, and ESSENCE. In addition, I shall try to provide helpful advice about possible approaches to intervention, and a basis for my own thoughts about how best to use the newly acquired information.

I would like to thank three people who have helped tremendously in the production of this book. Charles Olsen and Theo Gillberg translated into English a number of chapters and texts first drafted in Swedish. Without their help, the book would never have been completed. I am so grateful to both of you. Anna Spyrou proofread and corrected the final English draft and helped in a most professional and friendly way in the referencing and production of the list of references. Without your help I would not have been able to reach the final deadline.

Christopher Gillberg
June 2013

Introduction

Melchior Adam Weikard, physician to the Russian empress Catherine II, published a medical textbook that includes a chapter on "Attention Deficits" around 1770. The Scottish physician Alexander Crichton described attention deficits in young children in the 1790s (Crichton, 1798). He depicted a condition presenting in early childhood characterized by "incapacity of attending with a necessary degree of constancy, to any object." About 50 years later, extreme over-activity was described in certain children with epilepsy, and a children's story ("Fidgety Phil") was published that contained a literary portrait of a young boy who would definitely have been diagnosed with ADHD had he been seen by a child and adolescent psychiatrist or a pediatrician today (Hoffmann, 1845). Another 50 years later, the English pediatrician George Still described a condition in children that included emotional dysregulation, hyperactivity, lack of impulse control, and difficulties in concentration. He referred to the condition as a syndrome of "moral defect" (Still, 1902). About 20 years later it became clear that children could be affected by the kind of problems that Still had described in the aftermath of epidemic encephalitis. Since children who exhibited such symptoms after recovering from the acute effects of the hyperkinetic variant of so-called encephalitis lethargica (von Economo's encephalitis, also known as "sleepy sickness") generally seemed to be of average intelligence, one assumed that they had suffered a minimal brain injury (Gesell & Amatruda, 1947; Strauss & Lehtinen, 1947). This was probably how the controversial term MBD—short for minimal brain damage—was born (see Reid et al., 2001).

For several decades, the diagnosis of MBD was sporadically given to children who exhibited combinations of difficulties in socializing with peers and school adjustment and for whom motor overactivity was a cardinal symptom. Some of these were treated in the United States with stimulants following Charles Bradley's discovery during the 1930s that such treatment often lessened overactivity while simultaneously improving concentration.

Toward the end of the 1940s the term MBD or MBI (minimal brain injury) became even more topical due to the fact that overactivity was being described as a characteristic consequence of both traumatically and infectiously triggered brain damage (Gesell & Amatruda, 1947; Strauss & Lehtinen, 1947).

During the 1950s the term MBD became firmly rooted, especially in American child psychiatry and child neurology. Not least the British had doubts about using the term and organized a researcher convention in the early 1960s with the aim of "abolishing" MBD as a medical diagnosis. There was, however, a certain degree of dissension on the subject, and they only managed to change the meaning of the letter "D" in MBD. It was thus that minimal brain *dysfunction* came to replace minimal brain *damage*, and the term MBD remained for another 20 years—at least.

During the early 1980s the English child psychiatrist Michael Rutter wrote an influential paper in which he strongly contested the term MBD. He pointed to its irrationality in that (1) many children with the diagnosis MBD—with the methods available at the time—could not be proven to have any brain damage or brain disorder, (2) many children with proven brain damage did not have the type of problems that children with the diagnosis MBD exhibited, (3) some observations suggested that MBD could be a manifestation of widespread—and far from minimal—brain damage, (4) minimal brain damage could affect many different parts of the brain and the symptoms would then necessarily vary between different cases, and (5) other fields of child psychiatry/child neurology had avoided speculative "causal diagnoses" in favor of descriptive, neutral terms, and there was no reason why the MBD field should be any exception (Rutter, 1982). Rutter's paper marked the beginning of a more rational attitude toward the term MBD and it soon, certainly within the research community, fell into relative disuse. The term is still used in many parts of the world, although increasingly rarely. Within the research community, students of the condition instead refer to the symptoms and types of problems that the children exhibit, for example ADHD (attention-deficit/hyperactivity disorder), ADD (attention deficit disorder, often also referred to as inattentive subtype of ADHD), DAMP (deficits in attention, motor control, and perception), difficulties in concentration, impulse control problems, hyperactivity, HKD (hyperkinetic disorder), motor clumsiness, DCD (developmental coordination disorder), and intellectual disability or IDD (intellectual developmental disorder) (American Psychiatric Association, 1994, 2013; Gillberg, 1991).

Today, the term ADHD is definitely the predominant one in the whole field of attention disorders, even though the English "hyperkinetic disorder" (HKD) and the Nordic term DAMP are sometimes used as well. Both ADHD and particularly HKD are hampered by the fact that they include only a few of the types of problems that, for many of those affected, give rise to the most symptoms, nor do they refer in a comprehensive fashion to the ones that contribute to the long-term prognosis being very unfavorable in many cases. Motor control coordination problems, perception disorders, deficits in automation, and disorders affecting learning ability are all commonly, indeed almost universally, occurring among children and adolescents with early onset of difficulties in concentration. For this reason and because we do not yet know whether "attention problems," "hyperactivity," impulsivity, or the problems with motor control and perception are the most "core," some Nordic clinicians and researchers have preferred the term DAMP, which in itself includes several of the most important problem types. In recent years, the term ESSENCE has been launched. ESSENCE refers to Early Symptomatic Syndromes Eliciting Neurodevelopmental Clinical Examinations (Gillberg, 2010). It includes ADHD and all its many associated problems, including ASD, Tourette syndrome and other tic disorders, communication disorders, IDD, early-onset affective (including bipolar) disorders, and various types of behavioral and cognitive manifestations of underlying neurological (including epilepsy) and genetic disorders. It emphasizes that ADHD and the other types of problems included under the ESSENCE acronym only very rarely (if at all in the clinical world) exist without other problems and that coexistence of disorders ("comorbidity" to use a much-used misnomer phrase) *must* be anticipated and assessed for every time a child (or adult) comes to any kind of clinic with a named or suspected presenting symptom/disorder, be it ADHD, ASD, IDD, or other major developmental problem.

In this book the terms ADHD, DAMP, and ESSENCE will be the ones most often used. These are the terms that are now widespread in Sweden and other parts of Europe. DAMP is what best summarizes the complex constellation of difficulties that at least one child in every Scandinavian school class struggles with: attention deficit/activity control and impulse dysregulation, problems with motor control coordination (including motor expressive language), and difficulties in perception (including language/auditory reception). ADHD, on the other hand, is definitely the term predominantly used internationally. It refers to a large group of children with attention deficit/hyperactivity, many of whom have additional problems within the field of motor control and perception (and language) and hence meet the criteria for DAMP (Gillberg, 2003). ESSENCE is a concept that was launched officially only in 2010, but it has already gained substantial interest internationally.

In several chapters of this book reference will be made to the Gothenburg and other Scandinavian studies of ADHD and DAMP (corresponding to "comorbid" ADHD and DCD). These long-term, mostly Swedish, studies (about 60 altogether), along with a very large number of other international studies of ADHD (well over 40,000), form the basis for many of the conclusions presented in the book (Barkley, 2011; Biederman et al., 2011; Gillberg, 2003).

The Gothenburg total population longitudinal study of MBD/DAMP/ADHD started in the mid-1970s, at a time when MBD was still the term generally used (Gillberg, C., 1981; Gillberg, C., & Rasmussen, 1982; Gillberg,

I. C., 1987; Hellgren, 1994). It has therefore sometimes been referred to as the "MBD Study." Children born in 1969 and 1971 were examined at the age of 6 in preschool by their teachers who, by using a questionnaire, identified who probably had problems and who did not. Children from both these groups were then examined around the age of 7 by two child psychiatrists, a child neurologist, a psychologist, a neurophysiologist, and a physiotherapist. All the children were examined both in their home and at an outpatient clinic with a view to forming an opinion about whether or not their behavior and problems varied significantly between these different settings. The expert group performing the examinations had no knowledge of whether the preschool teachers had believed that the different individuals had a problem or not. Diagnoses of different kinds (for example, DAMP and ADHD) were made when the children were 7 years old. A follow-up of the group born in the 1971—both children with and without ADHD/DAMP—was then performed by expert groups who were not aware of the previous assessments at ages 10, 13, 16 to 17, and 22. None of the children in the study had been treated with stimulants. Such medication is prescribed at a very high rate in the United States, for example. Therefore, in this regard, the Swedish study provided a clearer view of the natural progression of ADHD/DAMP than a number of American studies do. One weakness of the study is the relatively small number of children with an ADHD/DAMP diagnosis (about 60 children), and about the same number of comparison cases (controls), who were observed over a 15-year period (Rasmussen & Gillberg, 2000). Several other important studies of ADHD/DAMP have been performed in the Nordic countries, and elsewhere in the world. These studies have confirmed the results of the Gothenburg study in many important respects, such as in terms of prevalence, correlation with other ESSENCE, and prognosis.

CONCLUDING REMARKS

ADHD, DAMP, and ESSENCE are relatively new terms that have replaced the term MBD, which over the 20th century had grown increasingly watered-down. In most of the world, the term ADHD is now used, although this emphasizes only one component—the attention deficit/ hyperactivity—in the complex of problems that characterize children with "MBD problems." Some U.K. specialists still prefer referring to HKD, but even in the United Kingdom ADHD/DAMP/ESSENCE has gained ground over the past several years. The diagnostic terms are numerous and confusing. In this book the terms ADHD, DAMP, and ESSENCE will be used most of the time since these acronyms—in a relatively neutral manner—describe the difficulties and categories of problems that affected children, adolescents, and adults struggle with.

REFERENCES

American Psychiatric Association (1994). *Diagnostic and statistical manual of mental disorders* (4th ed.). Washington, DC: APA.
American Psychiatric Association (2013). *Diagnostic and statistical manual of mental disorders* (5th ed.). Washington, DC: APA.
Barkley, R.A. (2011). Commentary on hyperkinetic impulse disorder. *Journal of Attention Disorders, 15,* 626–627.
Biederman, J., Petty, C.R., Clarke, A., Lomedico, A., & Faraone, S.V. (2011). Predictors of persistent ADHD: an 11-year follow-up study. *Journal of Psychiatric Research, 45,* 150–155.
Crichton, A. (1798). *An inquiry into the nature and origin of mental derangement: comprehending a concise system of the physiology and pathology of the human mind and a history of the passions and their effects.* Volume, 1. London: Cadell and Davies.
Gesell, A., & Amatruda, C.S. (1947). *Developmental diagnosis: normal and abnormal child development, clinical methods and pediatric applications* (2nd ed.). New York: Hoeber Publishing Co.
Gillberg, C. (1981). [Infantile autism—facts and fiction]. *Läkartidningen, 78,* 4373–4376.
Gillberg, C. (1991). [Scandinavian unity on MBD assessment. The term is old-fashioned and unsuitable]. *Läkartidningen, 88,* 713–714, 717.
Gillberg, C. (2003). Deficits in attention, motor control, and perception: a brief review. *Archives of Disease in Childhood, 88,* 904–910.
Gillberg, C. (2010). The ESSENCE in child psychiatry: early symptomatic syndromes eliciting neurodevelopmental clinical examinations. *Research in Developmental Disabilities, 31,* 1543–1551.
Gillberg, C., & Rasmussen, P. (1982). [A study in Gothenburg: minimal brain dysfunction in 6–7-year-old children can be traced by simple diagnostic aids]. *Läkartidningen, 79,* 4413–4414, 4419.

Gillberg, I.C. (1987). *Deficits in attention, motor control and perception: follow-up from pre-school to the early teens thesis*. (Doctoral Thesis). Uppsala University, Uppsala.

Hellgren, L. (1994). *Psychiatric disorders in adolescence. Longitudinal follow-up studies of adolescent onset psychoses and childhood onset deficits in attention motor control and perception*. (Doctoral Thesis). Gothenburg University, Gothenburg.

Hoffmann, H. (1995). *Struwwelpeter* (English translation). Mineola, NY: Dover. (Original work published 1845).

Rasmussen, P., & Gillberg, C. (2000). Natural outcome of ADHD with developmental coordination disorder at age 22 years: a controlled, longitudinal, community-based study. *Journal of the American Academy of Child and Adolescent Psychiatry*, *39*, 1424–1431.

Reid, A.H., McCall, S., Henry, J.M., & Taubenberger, J.K. (2001). Experimenting on the past: the enigma of von Economo's encephalitis lethargica. *Journal of Neuropathology and Experimental Neurology*, *60*, 663–670.

Rutter, M. (1982). Syndromes attributed to "minimal brain dysfunction" in childhood. *American Journal of Psychiatry*, *139*, 21–33.

Still, G.F. (1902). Some abnormal physical conditions in children: the Goulstonian lectures. *Lancet*, *1*, 1008–1012.

Strauss, A.A., & Lehtinen, L.E. (1947) *Psychopathology and education of the brain-injured child*. New York: Grune & Stratton.

Definitions and Diagnostic Criteria

Many of the most important terms and diagnostic categories used in this book will be defined in this chapter. The terms and categories are defined and delineated here and will henceforth be used with the assumption that the term/abbreviation/acronym is familiar to the reader.

As this book goes to press, the latest version of the American Psychiatric Association (APA)'s *Diagnostic and Statistical Manual of Mental Disorders* (the DSM-5) has just been released. Along with the International Classification of Diseases (ICD), it represents the best and most widely agreed-on information available for clinical diagnosis of neurodevelopmental or "neuropsychiatric" disorders. The DSM-5 will probably remain the key resource for delivering the best available clinical care for several years to come. This prognosis, to an extent, probably will fly in the face of accumulating evidence that clinically completely distinct disorders of neuropsychiatry do not exist, that they are the behavioral presentations of hundreds of different diseases or disorders, of amalgams of clinical spectra, and sometimes representations of the most extreme endpoints of "normal distribution."

Yet, what may be realistically feasible today for clinical practitioners will probably no longer be sufficient for researchers. The National Institute of Mental Health (NIMH) in the United States recently announced that in research, the categorical boundaries imposed by the exclusive use of categorical clinical concepts would no longer be accepted as a unique basis for delineating phenotypes in clinical research. Looking forward, laying the groundwork for a future diagnostic system that more directly reflects modern brain science will require openness to rethinking traditional categories. It is increasingly evident that mental illness will be best understood as disorders of brain structure and function that implicate specific domains of cognition, emotion, and behavior, domains that when tapped into will reveal, in most instances and in the majority of cases, a normal distribution or semi-normal distribution of functioning. To an extent, cutoff for disorder will always be arbitrary and may, in clinical practice, have less to do with the "correct" clinical phenotype than with factors associated with referral, degree of adaptive functioning, and associated problems not specifically relating to the spectrum of problems included under the particular diagnostic label.

The focus of this book is clearly clinical, and so categorical distinctions between disorders will be accepted as the clinical baseline. However, it should be clear to the reader that an absolutely clear-cut separation is usually not possible between case and non-case or between one named disorder and another. This stance will be clearly reflected in the following section on ESSENCE.

ESSENCE (EARLY SYMPTOMATIC SYNDROMES ELICITING NEURODEVELOPMENTAL CLINICAL EXAMINATIONS)

ESSENCE is an acronym launched in 2009 at the Royal College of Psychiatrists Annual Meeting in Liverpool by the author of this book. It stands for Early Symptomatic Syndromes Eliciting Neurodevelopmental Clinical Examinations (Gillberg, 2010). It covers ADHD and all the other early-onset neurodevelopmental/neuropsychiatric categorical "disorders" that it tends to be associated with (DCD, oppositional defiant disorder [ODD], autism spectrum disorder [ASD], tic disorders, speech and language disorders, and neurological disorders [including epilepsy] presenting with cognitive and/or behavioral symptoms at an early age). It refers to the reality of children (with their parents) presenting in clinical settings with impairing child symptoms before age 5 or 6 years in the fields of (a) general development, (b) communication and language, (c) social inter-relatedness, (d) motor coordination, (e) attention, (f) activity, (g) behavior, (h) mood, and/or (i) sleep/feeding. Children with major difficulties in one or more (usually several) of these fields will be referred to and assessed by health visitors, nurses, social workers, education specialists, pediatricians, GPs, speech and language therapists, child neurologists, child psychiatrists, psychologists, neurophysiologists, dentists, clinical geneticists, occupational therapists, and physiotherapists, but usually they will be seen by only one of these specialists when they would have needed the input of two or more of the experts referred to. The existence of major problems in at least one ESSENCE domain before age 6 years often signals major problems in the same or overlapping domains years later. Most of the disorders subsumed under ESSENCE occur at a rate of about 1% or more of the general population, with ADHD, affecting about 5%, being the most common. Because of the extreme degree of overlap between these clinically delineated disorders, the total rate for all ESSENCE is much lower than would be expected if we were only to sum up all the prevalence rates listed, but still at a rate of almost 10% of the whole child population. See more about ESSENCE in Chapter 3.

ADHD (ATTENTION-DEFICIT/HYPERACTIVITY DISORDER)

ADHD refers to a condition present from childhood and with clear problems presenting within the areas of attention, (hyper) activity, and/or impulsiveness (Table 2.1). The clinical presentation is one that is consistent with the criteria found in the DSM-IV (APA, 1994) and the DSM-5 (APA, 2013) and overlapping with (but not identical to) that described as hyperkinetic disorder (HKD) (see below) in the ICD-10 (WHO, 1993) and ICD-11 (WHO, in progress). Three different types of ADHD were first described and coded separately in the DSM-IV, and these subtypes are retained under the DSM-5. The three subtypes appear to have some clinical face validity, although it is possible that only the last two in Table 2.1 are usually associated with moderate to severe functional disability, while the first one appears to have much more variable clinical impairment:

1. ADHD dominated by hyperactivity and lack of impulse control, referred to as **ADHD, predominantly hyperactive-impulsive subtype**
2. ADHD dominated by attention deficit, referred to as *ADHD, predominantly inattentive subtype* (also now sometimes referred to as ADD, see below)
3. ADHD, combined form with both attention deficit and hyperactivity/lack of impulse control, referred to as **ADHD, combined subtype.**

Some recent studies suggest that the underlying factor structure of ADHD is that of an attention deficit on the one hand and a lack of impulse control on the other (Ullebø et al., 2012) and that the matter of hyperactivity has come to be overrated in the context of ADHD symptomatology. There are certainly children and adults who are very active ("hyperactive"?) but who show few, if any, signs of inattention or impulsivity. Even when they meet symptom criteria for ADHD, it is doubtful whether they should be given a diagnosis of the disorder. Most recent prevalence studies actually suggest that the "pure" hyperactive subtype of ADHD is very rare and that the inattention and combined subtypes are much more common.

According to the DSM-5, an ADHD diagnosis can be assigned regardless of IQ (see below) and the presence or not of any additional physical or psychiatric diagnosis or problem. In previous versions of the DSM (DSM-IV and DSM-IV-TR/Text Revision) (APA, 2000), certain exclusionary criteria were specified, and most researchers and clinicians interpreted these to mean that ADHD could not be diagnosed, for instance, in association with autism. Research in recent years has shown convincingly that ADHD symptom criteria are often met in autism and other autism spectrum disorders and that autistic features are very often present in

TABLE 2.1.
ADHD ACCORDING TO DSM-5 (SYMPTOM CRITERIA GENERALLY
CONSISTENT WITH DSM-IV)

A. Either A.1 or A.2:
A1. Inattention: Six (or more) of the following nine symptoms have persisted for at least 6 months to a degree that is inconsistent with developmental level and that impact directly on social and academic/occupational activities.
a. Often fails to give close attention to details or makes careless mistakes in schoolwork, at work, or during other activities (e.g., overlooks or misses details, work is inaccurate).
b. Often has difficulty sustaining attention in tasks or play activities (e.g., has difficulty remaining focused during lectures, conversations, or reading lengthy writings).
c. Often does not seem to listen when spoken to directly (e.g., mind seems elsewhere, even in the absence of any obvious distraction).
d. Often does not follow through on instructions and fails to finish schoolwork, chores, or duties in the workplace (e.g., starts tasks but quickly loses focus and is easily sidetracked; fails to finish schoolwork, household chores, or tasks in the workplace).
e. Often has difficulty organizing tasks and activities (e.g., difficulty managing sequential tasks; difficulty keeping materials and belongings in order; messy, disorganized, work; poor time management; tends to fail to meet deadlines).
f. Often avoids, dislikes, or is reluctant to engage in tasks that require sustained mental effort (e.g., schoolwork or homework; for older adolescents and adults, preparing reports, completing forms, or reviewing lengthy papers).
g. Often loses things necessary for tasks or activities (e.g., school materials, pencils, books, tools, wallets, keys, paperwork, eyeglasses, or mobile telephones).
h. Is often easily distracted by extraneous stimuli (for older adolescents and adults, may include unrelated thoughts).
i. Is often forgetful in daily activities (e.g., chores, running errands; for older adolescents and adults, returning calls, paying bills, keeping appointments).
A2. Hyperactivity and Impulsivity: Six (or more) of the following symptoms have persisted for at least 6 months to a degree that is inconsistent with developmental level and that impact directly on social and academic/ occupational activities.

TABLE 2.1.
(CONTINUED)

a. Often fidgets with or taps hands or feet or squirms in seat.
b. Often leaves seat in situations when remaining seated is expected (e.g., leaves his or her place in the classroom, office or other workplace, or in other situations that require remaining seated).
c. Often runs about or climbs in situations where it is inappropriate. (In adolescents or adults, may be limited to feeling restless).
d. Often unable to play or engage in leisure activities quietly.
e. Is often "on the go," acting as if "driven by a motor" (e.g., is unable or uncomfortable being still for an extended time, as in restaurants, meetings, etc; may be experienced by others as being restless and difficult to keep up with).
f. Often talks excessively.
g. Often blurts out an answer before a question has been completed (e.g., completes people's sentences and "jumps the gun" in conversations, cannot wait for next turn in conversation).
h. Often has difficulty waiting his or her turn (e.g., while waiting in line).
i. Often interrupts or intrudes on others (e.g., butts into conversations, games, or activities; may start using other people's things without asking or receiving permission, adolescents or adults may intrude into or take over what others are doing).
B. Several inattentive or hyperactive-impulsive symptoms were present prior to age 12 (7 under DSM-IV).
C. Criteria for the disorder are met in two or more settings (e.g., at home, school or work, with friends or relatives, or in other activities).
D. There must be clear evidence that the symptoms interfere with or reduce the quality of social, academic, or occupational functioning.
E. The symptoms do not occur exclusively during the course of schizophrenia or another psychotic disorder and are not better accounted for by another mental disorder (e.g., mood disorder, anxiety disorder, dissociative disorder, or a personality disorder).
Specify Based on Current Presentation
Combined Presentation: If both Criterion A1 (Inattention) and Criterion A2 (Hyperactivity-Impulsivity) are met for the past 6 months.

(continued)

TABLE 2.1.
(CONTINUED)

Predominantly Inattentive Presentation: If Criterion A1 (Inattention) is met but Criterion A2 (Hyperactivity-Impulsivity) is not met and 3 or more symptoms from Criterion A2 have been present for the past 6 months.
Inattentive Presentation (Restrictive): If Criterion A1 (Inattention) is met but no more than 2 symptoms from Criterion A2 (Hyperactivity-Impulsivity) have been present for the past 6 months.
Predominantly Hyperactive/Impulsive Presentation: If Criterion A2 (Hyperactivity-Impulsivity) is met and Criterion A1 (Inattention) is not met for the past 6 months.
Coding note: For individuals (especially adolescents and adults) who currently have symptoms with impairment that no longer meet full criteria, "In Partial Remission" should be specified.

Reprinted with permission from the Diagnostic and Statistical Manual of Mental Disorders, Fifth Edition, (Copyright 2013). American Psychiatric Association.

young people meeting diagnostic criteria for ADHD (Kopp et al., 2010; Lundström et al., 2011).

Around half of all children with ADHD also meet the full criteria for DCD and therefore, by definition, also those of DAMP (see below). About half of all children diagnosed with ADHD have too few symptoms of motor control/perception problems (DCD-type difficulties) for a DCD/DAMP diagnosis to be given, which does not mean that this "non-DCD group" is completely free of motor-perceptual problems (Kadesjö & Gillberg, 1999). Instead, it is likely that the vast majority of individuals with ADHD also have some motor control problems. It is unclear whether the motor problems should be regarded as completely separate or a result of underlying executive function deficits (see this term) leading to difficulties controlling attention, impulses, activity, *and* motor functioning. There is no consensus in this field at the present time. What is clear, though, is that motor control problems are grossly underrated as a cause of suffering in ADHD.

One difficulty with the ADHD concept is that it implies that hyperactivity is a given part of the problem, and one that is crucial for the diagnosis to be made. There are, however, many people with ADHD who are not "overtly" hyperactive, and a smaller group that actually would have to be described as hypoactive. The insight into these problems surrounding the diagnostic term itself has led to the addition of a forward slash sign between "attention-deficit" and "hyperactivity disorder" in the DSM-IV and the DSM-5 (something that was not present in DSM-III-R, the predecessor of DSM-IV). The slash sign indicates that the problem can be either "AD" or "HD"—or both. As has already been alluded to, recent studies suggest that the two independent factors within the ADHD "phenotype" are inattention and impulsivity, rather than hyperactivity.

ADD (ATTENTION-DEFICIT DISORDER)

In the past, the whole ADHD "group" was, for a time, referred to as ADD. When the ADD term is used today it often refers to ADHD dominated by attention deficit.

Nowadays, when ADD is discussed as a clinical concept or a separate diagnosis, it is usually synonymous with ADHD, mainly inattentive subtype. Given that most individuals with this variant ("ADD") are not at all hyperactive or even impulsive, the link with "ADHD" (often perceived as being symptomatically dominated by hyperactive-impulsive behavior) may appear tenuous. Nevertheless, there is clearly a group of individuals within the broader ADHD group in whom inattention problems are very striking, processing is often slow, and there is a general impression of sluggish tempo, and it is often to this group that the label of ADD is applied.

HKD (HYPERKINETIC DISORDER)

In the United Kingdom, the term HKD (hyperkinetic disorder)—from the ICD-10—is still often used, but in most other countries it is considered obsolete. It refers to a large subgroup of the patients who have "combined ADHD," namely those who have attention deficit *and* hyperactivity *and* impulsivity and are severely handicapped by these problems in most situations in everyday life. It is sometimes portrayed as the "clinically meaningful" variant of ADHD and the one that most predictably will respond to stimulant medication (Banaschewski et al., 2006). However, the research specifically related to the syndrome delineated in the ICD-10 is very limited and cannot even begin to compare with the amount of study that has been devoted specifically to the DSM category of ADHD.

DCD/MPD (DEVELOPMENTAL COORDINATION DISORDER/MOTOR PERCEPTION DYSFUNCTION)

MPD—now more often collectively referred to as DCD—refers to the presence of difficulties in motor control and/or problems with perception that are clearly more pronounced than expected for chronological or developmental age and that can be documented through a medical examination and/or neurological testing. The dysfunction is diagnosed only if the individual is clearly impaired in everyday functioning. Some specialists, perhaps particularly occupational therapists and speech and language pathology therapists, use the term "dyspraxia" to cover many of the symptoms shown by children who have DCD.

DCD is the near-synonym of MPD in the DSM. The problems in perception are not emphasized under this diagnosis but are most likely significant in the majority of all patients with DCD (APA, 2013; Kadesjö & Gillberg, 1999).

DCD is part and parcel of a number of conditions/disorders subsumed under the ESSENCE umbrella. It is commonly encountered in children with a "primary" diagnosis of ADHD and/or ASD. However, it is still often missed as a separate problem category and very often overlooked when it comes to intervention programs or educational plans.

DAMP (DEFICITS IN ATTENTION, MOTOR CONTROL, AND PERCEPTION)

A Nordic expert group agreed in 1990 to use the term DAMP instead of MBD (Airaksinen et al., 1991). DAMP, in more modern terminology, is the combination of ADHD and DCD (Gillberg, 2003). The term is little used outside of the Nordic countries.

All individuals with DAMP have difficulties in activity control and attention (corresponding to ADHD any subtype) *and* problems with motor control/perception (mirroring those found in DCD) (Table 2.2). In other words, DAMP constitutes a large subgroup among all individuals who meet the criteria for ADHD. Activity control and attention are always problematic, but the difficulties within the motor and perceptual spectrum can pertain to *either* motor control *or* perception. In practice, however, the case is virtually always that, if there are considerable difficulties in perception, there are also problems with motor control present. In brief, all people clinically diagnosed with DAMP have problems with activity control and/or attention combined with difficulties in motor control. About two out of three of these have perception disorders in addition to the other problems.

The difficulties in activity control and attention must be possible to document in several different situations, for example both at home and in school, and meet the criteria for one of the DSM variants of ADHD. Hyperactivity, hypoactivity, and combinations of these (alternating between hyper- and hypoactivity) are prevalent. Fewer than half of all children in the DAMP group are severely hyperactive. However, they all have difficulties adjusting their activity level to what is required of the present situation, and they all have marked attention difficulties.

For a diagnosis of DAMP (which is not listed in the DSM or ICD but corresponds to DSM "ADHD with DCD"), difficulties in motor control must—at least if the child has reached the age of around 5to 8 years of age—be possible to document through a medical examination. If the child is younger than 5 years, there must be some evidence of clumsy motor control or of abnormal expressive speech development, which, in this context, is considered a symptom of abnormal motor control. If the child is older, there can be considerable abnormalities at the time of the medical examination, previously documented abnormalities, an overall clinical gestalt of clumsy and ill-coordinated body movements, or a strong conviction in the older individual himself herself of motor clumsiness (that

TABLE 2.2.
DIAGNOSTIC CRITERIA FOR DAMP

Symptom Area	Diagnostic Delimitation
A. Activity control	ADHD according to DSM-5
	Severe problems (in several different situations) if all of the following are present:
	(1) activity control (hyper- or hypoactivity or both)
	(2) ability to concentrate
	(3) attention
	(4) ability to stay still
	Moderate problems (in several different situations) if two or three of (1), (2), (3), and (4) are present.
B. Motor control	DCD according to DSM-5, i.e. in practice considerable difficulties in gross or fine motor skills
C. Perception	Considerable difficulties in visual perception according to generally recognized tests as described by Gillberg et al.[1] and Landgren et al.[2]; usually corresponding to or "comorbid with" DSM-5 DCD

Diagnosis of DAMP requires that both A and B apply (i.e., A. ADHD according to DSM-5 and B. DCD according to DSM-5). These criteria are according to Gillberg et al. (1982),[1] updated by Landgren et al. (1996)[2] and revised by Kadesjö & Gillberg (1998)[3]: updated for the publication of this book by the author (2013).

[1]Gillberg, C., Rasmussen, P., Carlström, G., Svensson, B., & Waldenström, E. (1982). Perceptual, motor and attentional deficits in six-year-old children. Epidemiological aspects. *Journal of Child Psychology and Psychiatry, 23*, 131–144.

[2]Landgren, Petterson, R., Kjellman, B., & Gillberg, C. (1996). ADHD, DAMP and other neurodevelopmental/psychiatric disorders in six-year-old children. Epidemiology and comorbidity. *Developmental Medicine and Child Neurology, 38*, 891–906.

[3]Kadesjö, B., & Gillberg, C. (1998). Attention deficits and clumsiness in Swedish 7-year-old children. *Developmental Medicine and Child Neurology, 40*, 796–811.

[4]Rasmussen, P., Gillberg, C., Waldenström, E., & Svenson, B. (1983). Perceptual, motor and attentional deficits in seven-year-old children. Neurological and neurodevelopmental aspects. *Developmental Medicine and Child Neurology, 25*, 315–333.

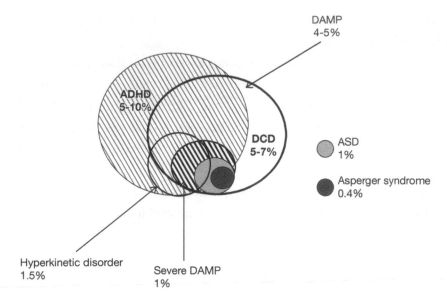

Figure 2.1.
The overlap of attention deficits and DCD. Figure drawn by C. Gillberg.

---

is not clearly contradicted by actual testing), even when brief examination no longer conclusively supports the presence of a motor/neurological abnormality. The motor abnormalities can affect gross motor skills (large physical movements) or fine motor skills (primarily manual and oral motor skills), usually both. One is usually able to demonstrate the difficulties in perception through abnormal results on neuropsychological tests, such as several of those reflecting "perceptual organization" on the Wechsler scales. These results can usually be matched by the descriptions of a variety of different symptoms of perceptual difficulties.

The neuropsychological test profile in cases of DAMP is usually uneven. In terms of "learning," about 20% of all children, adolescents, and adults with the condition function at the same level as—or almost at the same level as—individuals with intellectual disability/IDD (see below)—that is, at "special school" level. A clinical DAMP diagnosis should not be made if the intelligence profile is even/smooth and it is apparent that there is an intellectual impairment with an IQ below 70, and the "IDD as such" is the best explanation for the child's symptoms. In practice, though, it can be difficult to determine whether the main diagnosis should be DAMP or mild intellectual disability.

In about 20% of cases of DAMP motor control is so abnormal that the diagnosis "mild cerebral palsy" (Rasmussen et al., 1983) might come under consideration. In principle, however, the clinical diagnosis of DAMP should not be made if it is obvious that cerebral palsy is present. However, a diagnosis of ADHD (without DCD) may, nevertheless, be appropriate in some such cases.

DAMP is sometimes split into two groups: severe DAMP and moderate DAMP. Severe DAMP means that there are problems within all of the following five areas:

1. Activity-impulsivity and/or attention
2. Gross motor skills
3. Fine motor skills
4. Perception
5. Language and speech

Moderate DAMP means that there are difficulties in area (1) in combination with problems within one, two, or three (but not all four) of the other areas.

These two definitions together mean that all patients who meet the general criteria for DAMP (i.e., ADHD with DCD) and do not meet the criteria for severe DAMP (i.e., that the problems exist within all areas listed under (1) through (5) above) should be diagnosed with moderate DAMP.

Again, it needs emphasizing that DAMP is not a diagnosis that is officially recognized in the currently most used diagnostic systems (ICD or DSM). Nevertheless, it refers to an entity that is well recognized by clinicians who have worked with children with neurodevelopmental disorders for a long period of time. If one concentrates all one's diagnostic efforts on the attention/activity/impulsivity problems inherent in ADHD, the very significant motor-perceptual problems that so many of the children with ADHD suffer from may well be (and are often) missed. The DAMP construct, as we shall see, has advantages in that it takes account of a much broader range of problems, including also language/communication problems, that are the clinical rule in the vast majority of patients with "ADHD" (Gillberg, 2003; Sturm et al., 2004).

IQ, BIF (BORDERLINE INTELLECTUAL FUNCTIONING), AND IDD (INTELLECTUAL DEVELOPMENTAL DISORDER)

In clinical child practice, IQ refers to a figure that states what percentage the individual has of the average level of intelligence within a certain age group. A 10-year-old with an IQ of 80 has 80% of the average intelligence of all 10-year-olds. His or her intellectual function would then be 80% of that of an average 10-year-old, and thus he or she functions at the level of an 8-year-old (80% of 10 years equals 8 years). A 10-year-old with an IQ of 120 functions at a level equal to that of a 12-year-old (120% of 10 years equals 12 years).

If a person's IQ is between around 70 and 85, then that is referred to as borderline intelligence or BIF. If a person's IQ is above 115, then that it is referred to as above-average intelligence. IQ of above around 130 is considered exceptional intelligence.

IDD (previously mental retardation) refers to the presence of an intellectual impairment that is apparent at an early age and that is usually of prenatal origin or acquired during the first years of life. IQ is equal to or below circa 70. The individual needs significant educational and other supportive measures; that is, he or she has markedly reduced adaptive abilities. The diagnosis is clinical and not based solely on the result of one IQ test.

Mild IDD (special school level, "ESN school") is present if the individual has an IQ of around 50 to 70 (and a corresponding level of adaptive functioning). Moderate to severe IDD (training school level) is present if the person has an IQ below 50. Under the DSM-5, the severity level is determined more by the adaptive functioning than by the exact IQ level (even if the two are closely related in many cases).

The term "mental retardation" is outdated and should not be used in clinical practice. It is mentioned here just so that it may be obvious that IDD is "modern terminology" for exactly the same type of problem referred to in a huge body of older research as mental retardation.

NVLD/NLD (NONVERBAL LEARNING DISABILITY)

Some children and adults score relatively (or sometimes very) high on verbal tests and yet perform poorly (very or relatively) on the nonverbal ("performance") parts of IQ tests. When the discrepancy is great (with a difference of 15 to 25 points or more) and the individual is impaired in social or academic functioning, a diagnosis of NVLD or NLD may be warranted (Rourke, 1988, 2008). Individuals with this type of discrepancy are often socially impaired in ways that suggest autistic features (and primary or additional diagnoses of autism spectrum disorder, including Asperger syndrome, are often made). NVLD is not a diagnostic category in the DSM or ICD classification systems and should be seen as a neuropsychological diagnosis along the lines of "working memory disorder" or "slow processing disorder."

DYSLEXIA, READING AND WRITING DISORDER, AND DYSCALCULIA

Dyslexia, or "specific" difficulties in reading and writing (also referred to as reading disorder, sometimes nonspecifically lumped with writing disorder), refers to difficulties in reading (and writing) that cannot be explained by low IQ or the lack of sufficient social or educational stimuli. There must—according to the DSM—be a significant discrepancy between the person's ability to read and write on the one hand and his or her IQ on the other. This means that people with IDD can have dyslexia, but in such cases the ability to read and write is far below what might be expected given the person's IQ. It is hardly meaningful to discuss dyslexia in people with severe mental retardation (i.e., whose IQ is below 50), since the majority of them cannot be expected to learn how to read or write. On the other hand, dyslexia may very well present in someone with an average reading and/or writing ability and an IQ of 140. In such a person one would have, if dyslexia had not been involved, expected a reading/writing ability far above that of the average person. Some authors refer to dyslexia in cases of difficulties in reading and writing without any regard to IQ.

Dyscalculia, or "specific" difficulties with numbers and mathematical concepts and operations (sometimes also referred to as mathematics disorder), is the term used for difficulties with math/arithmetic that cannot be explained by low IQ or lack of sufficient social or educational stimuli. There is considerable overlap between dyslexia and dyscalculia, but the latter "specific" type of problem (i.e., when math problems are not associated with generally lower cognitive abilities) is rarer, particularly relatively rarer in boys.

CEREBRAL PALSY

Cerebral palsy is present in individuals who have a congenital, usually non-progressive, motor impairment with significant inhibition of their mobility. The causes are genetic and other disorders and injuries to the central nervous system that are either inherited or acquired at an early stage of development. There are different types of cerebral palsy, for example hemiplegia (unilateral poor motor function), diplegia (poor motor function primarily in both legs), tetraplegia (severely deficient motor function in all four extremities), and ataxia (lowered ability to coordinate motions with, for example, deficits in hand motor skills and balance). The types of motor dysfunction are related to the stage of brain development at the time of the occurrence of the adverse event-be it genetic or acquired (Bax et al., 2005).

MENTAL HEALTH DISORDERS/PSYCHIATRIC DISORDERS

A mental health disorder (psychiatric disorder/problem) is present in an individual with mental symptoms that cause considerable suffering either for the individual or for the people around him or her. One generally refers to it as a *disorder* only if the condition has lasted for a certain amount of time, for example longer than a week or a month or several months. Sometimes a line is drawn between a temporary mental disorder (psychiatric "state," such as occurs with acute anxiety, depression, or mania) and a psychiatric disability/psychiatric "trait" (such as in the case of borderline or antisocial personality disorder), which usually means that the "disorder" has existed for about six months or (much) longer.

Mental disorders can be classified in many different ways and divided into many subgroups. The DSM lists symptom criteria for a large number of psychiatric conditions, for example depression, bipolar disorder, separation anxiety disorder, generalized anxiety disorder, different types of personality disorder, and all the disorders with onset of symptoms in childhood, including conduct disorder, ODD, Asperger syndrome and other ASD, obsessive-compulsive disorder, and Tourette syndrome, to name only a few of the diagnoses that relatively often occur as associated problems in cases of ESSENCE/ADHD/DAMP.

CONCLUDING REMARKS

ADHD and DAMP (and indeed ESSENCE) are partly overlapping terms. Which of the "diagnoses" is given depends to some extent on where in the world the child or adult becomes the subject of examination. The terms are not synonymous: DAMP emphasizes the simultaneous occurrence of ADHD and DCD (motor/perceptual problems), whereas the diagnosis of ADHD focuses only on the attention deficit/hyperactivity.

In virtually all cases of impairing ADHD there are associated other problems, particularly learning difficulties, language problems, difficulties with reading and writing, and mental disorders (including emotional dyscontrol, oppositional defiant disorder, and oppositional defiant behaviors, conduct disorder, autistic features, tics, depression, and anxiety). One can have an adequate understanding of children, adolescents, and adults with ADHD/DAMP/ESSENCE only if one is also aware of these connections and so-called comorbidities.

REFERENCES

Airaksinen, E., Bille, B., Carlström, G., Diderichsen, J., Ehlers, S., Gillberg, C., et al. (1991). [Children and adolescents with DAMP/MBD]. *Läkartidningen, 88*, 714.

Aicardi, J., Bax, M., Gillberg, C. (Eds.). (2009). *Diseases of the nervous system in childhood* (3rd ed.). London: Mac Keith Press.

American Psychiatric Association (1994). *Diagnostic and statistical manual of mental disorders* (4th ed.) Washington, DC: APA.

American Psychiatric Association (2000). *Diagnostic and statistical manual of mental disorders*. (4th ed., text revision). Washington, DC: APA.

American Psychiatric Association (2013). *Diagnostic and statistical manual of mental disorders* (5th ed.). Washington, DC: APA.

Banaschewski, T., Coghill, D., Santosh, P., Zuddas, A., Asherson, P., Buitelaar, J., et al. (2006) Long-acting medications for the hyperkinetic disorders. A systematic review and European treatment guideline. *European Child & Adolescent Psychiatry, 15,* 476–495.

Bax, M., Goldstein, M., Rosenbaum, P., Leviton, A., Paneth, N., Dan, B. et al. (2005) Proposed definition and classification of cerebral palsy, April 2005. *Developmental Medicine and Child Neurology, 47,* 571–576.

Biederman, J., Mick, E., Faraone, S.V., Spencer, T., Wilens, T.E., & Wozniak, J. (2003). Current concepts in the validity, diagnosis and treatment of paediatric bipolar disorder. *International Journal of Neuropsychopharmacology, 6,* 293–300.

Coleman, M., & Gillberg, C. (2012). *The autisms* (4th ed.). New York: Oxford University Press.

Comings, D.E. (1990). *Tourette syndrome and human behaviour*. Duarte, CA: Hope Press.

Gillberg, C. (1995). *Clinical child neuropsychiatry*. Cambridge: Cambridge University Press.

Gillberg, C. (2003). Deficits in attention, motor control, and perception: a brief review. *Archives of Disease in Childhood, 88,* 904–910.

Gillberg, C. (2010). The ESSENCE in child psychiatry: early symptomatic syndromes eliciting neurodevelopmental clinical examinations. *Research in Developmental Disabilities, 31,* 1543–1551.

Gillberg, C., & Söderström, H. (2003). Learning disability. *Lancet, 362,* 811–821.

Kadesjö, B., & Gillberg, C. (1999). Developmental coordination disorder in Swedish 7-year-old children. *Journal of the American Academy of Child and Adolescent Psychiatry, 38,* 820–828.

Kopp, S., Kelly, K. B., & Gillberg, C. (2010). Girls with social and/or attention deficits: a descriptive study of 100 clinic attenders. *Journal of Attention Disorders, 14,* 167–181.

Lundström, S., Chang, Z., Kerekes, N., Gumpert, C.H., Råstam, M., Gillberg, C., et al. (2011). Autistic-like traits and their association with mental health problems in two nationwide twin cohorts of children and adults. *Psychological Medicine, 41,* 2423–2433.

Miniscalco, C., Nygren, G., Hagberg, B., Kadesjö, B., & Gillberg, C. (2006). Neuropsychiatric and neurodevelopmental outcome of children at age 6 and 7 years who screened positive for language problems at 30 months. *Developmental Medicine and Child Neurology, 48*, 361–366.

O'Brien, G. (2000). Behavioural phenotypes. *Journal of the Royal Society of Medicine, 93*, 618–620.

Pliszka, S.R. (2000). Patterns of psychiatric comorbidity with attention-deficit/hyperactivity disorder. *Child and Adolescent Psychiatric Clinics of North America, 9*, 525–540.

Rasmussen, P., Gillberg, C., Waldenström, E., & Svenson, B. (1983). Perceptual, motor and attentional deficits in seven-year-old children: neurological and neurodevelopmental aspects. *Developmental Medicine and Child Neurology, 25*, 315–333.

Rourke, B.P. (1988). The syndrome of nonverbal learning disabilities: Developmental manifestations in neurological disease, disorder, and dysfunction. *Clinical Neuropsychologist, 2*, 293–330.

Rourke, B.P. (2008). Is neuropsychology a psychosocial science? *Journal of Clinical and Experimental Neuropsychology, 30*, 691–699.

Sadiq, F.A., Slator, L., Skuse, D., Law, J., Gillberg, C., & Minnis, H. (2012). Social use of language in children with reactive attachment disorder and autism spectrum disorders. *European Child & Adolescent Psychiatry, 21*, 267–276.

Sturm, H., Fernell, E., & Gillberg, C. (2004). Autism spectrum disorders in children with normal intellectual levels: associated impairments and subgroups. *Developmental Medicine and Child Neurology, 46*, 444–447.

Swanson, J.M., Wigal, T., & Lakes, K. (2009). DSM-V and the future diagnosis of attention-deficit/hyperactivity disorder. *Current Psychiatry Reports, 11*, 399–406.

Ullebø, A.K., Breivik, K., Gillberg, C., Lundervold, A.J., & Posserud, M.B. (2012). The factor structure of ADHD in a general population of primary school children. *Journal of Child Psychology and Psychiatry, 53*, 927–936.

WHO (World Health Organization) (1993). *The ICD-10 classification of mental and behavioural disorders. Diagnostic criteria for research.* Geneva: WHO.

WHO (World Health Organization) (forthcoming, 2015). *The ICD-10 classification of mental and behavioural disorders. Diagnostic criteria for research.*

ADHD and the Concept of ESSENCE (Early Symptomatic Syndromes Eliciting Neurodevelopmental Clinical Examinations)

INTRODUCTION

ADHD is listed in the DSM-IV as a psychiatric disorder with onset in childhood. In the DSM-5 it is listed among neurodevelopmental disorders. Debate sometimes gets heated about whether or not it should be considered a "psychiatric," "neuropsychiatric," or "neurodevelopmental" disorder. Depending on the definitions of these three concepts, ADHD, of course, is well placed within all three categories. Debate also sometimes centers around whether or not ADHD is a "discrete categorical" disorder or a "dimensional" disorder, and also whether or not it can occur together with other conditions or disorders. The most reasonable answer to these three questions is "yes": ADHD can be separated out as a categorical disorder, it can be construed as one of the end sections on a dimension of

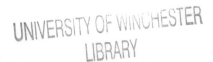

attention (or for that matter on a dimension of impulsivity), and it can definitely occur together with other problems. Indeed, almost all the epidemiological evidence relating to ADHD indicates that it is almost never an isolated disorder or collection of symptoms.

While in the past child psychiatry showed little interest in operationalized diagnosis, in recent times categorical diagnosis has become an integral part of everyday clinical and research practice. We are now so insistent on the distinction between "disorder" and "not disorder" ("normalcy") that clinics and clinicians become more and more specialized and cater to the needs of children with "attention-deficit/hyperactivity disorder/ADHD only," "autism only," or "Tourette syndrome only." This has led to a situation in which the typical clinical diffuseness of disorder has come to be underestimated.

At the same time, rather belatedly, there is growing acceptance that coexistence of disorders and sharing of symptoms across disorders (so-called comorbidity, a misnomer if ever there was one, seeing as we are usually not dealing with completely separate coexisting disorders) is the rule rather than the exception (e.g., Kadesjö & Gillberg 2001). This was pointed out more than a quarter of a century ago (Gillberg, 1983), but, in clinical practice, this insight has not led to new approaches when trying to address the needs of children and families with "complex needs." Instead, diversification has boomed.

There are legislational, scientific, and clinical attempts to separate out children with certain disorders/diagnoses (e.g., IDD and ASD) from those who do not meet the criteria for the disorder/diagnoses, all aiming to provide better societal guidelines, more focused attempts at finding the causes, and more specific services. Children with ADHD are targeted in similar ways, even though legislation has yet to catch up with them. The same holds for children with language impairments (often erroneously referred to as "specific" language impairment [SLI]—erroneous because the impairments are only very rarely specific), visual impairments, and hearing deficits (children who may, or may not, have additional impairments as regards general cognition, motor performance, ADHD, or ASD).

ADHD and ASD, which were long treated as and believed to be completely separate and recognizable "disorders," are now increasingly often diagnosed "together" within one and the same individual, and there is growing awareness that they sometimes overlap and constitute amalgams of problems, and that in some families they separate together and probably represent different aspects of the same underlying disorder (Constantino et al., 2007).

With increased understanding that early-onset childhood problems, such as those reflected in children who are diagnosed in the preschool or early school years as suffering from ADHD or ASD, have long-term, indeed probably often lifetime, consequences (Billstedt et al., 2005; Cederlund et al., 2010; Rasmussen & Gillberg, 2000), the incentives to screen and to diagnose these conditions have become main priorities for clinicians and administrators hoping to alter the often negative outcome typically seen in patients who have had little or no intervention (or indeed an exclusionary attitude on the part of those "responsible") during the course of growing up. The question to be addressed is this: Would making discrete diagnosis (of, say, ADHD or ASD) before age 5 to 6 years contribute to a better understanding, better intervention, and more positive outcomes in children who present with problems that could be indices of these disorders?

WHAT IS ESSENCE?

The acronym ESSENCE refers to Early Symptomatic Syndromes Sliciting Neurodevelopmental Clinical Examinations. It was coined with a view to highlighting the clinical reality of children (and their parents) presenting in first-, second-, or third-tier clinical settings with usually complex, impairing developmental symptoms before age 5 to 6 years. The children are reported to have problems in the fields of (a) general development, (b) communication and language, (c) social inter-relatedness, (d) motor coordination, (e) attention/" listening," (f) activity, (g) behavior, (h) mood, and/or (i) sleep. Children with major difficulties in one or more (usually several) of these fields will be referred to and seen by health visitors, nurses, social workers, education (including preschool) specialists, pediatricians, GPs, speech and language therapists, child neurologists, child psychiatrists, psychologists, neurophysiologists, dentists, clinical geneticists, occupational therapists, and physiotherapists, but in the vast majority of cases they will be seen by only one of these specialists when, in fact, they would have needed the input of two or more (occasionally even all) of the "experts" referred to.

The syndromes encompassed under the ESSENCE umbrella acronym are listed in Table 3.1.

Most of these syndromes are conceptualized as more or less discrete disorders in the DSM and ICD. Here they are listed, not because they are conceptualized as existing "in their own right" (even though occasionally they do show up as isolated conditions in individuals), but because

TABLE 3.1.
ESSENCE (I.E., NEURODEVELOPMENTAL SYNDROMES/DISORDERS USUALLY MANIFESTING WITH CLINICAL SYMPTOMS LEADING TO REFERRAL OR ASSESSMENT BEFORE ABOUT 6 YEARS OF AGE)

Syndrome	Prevalence	Key Reference
ADHD	5%	Swanson et al., 2009
DCD	5%	Kadesjö & Gillberg, 1999
ODD/Disruptive mood dysregulation	4%	Pliszka, 2000; Copeland et al., 2013
Tic disorders/Tourette syndrome	1%	Comings, 1990
ASD	1%	Coleman & Gillberg, 2012
Language disorder	4%	Miniscalco et al., 2006
IDD	1.5%	Gillberg & Söderström, 2003
NVLD	Unknown	Rourke, 1988
Bipolar disorder and major depression	Rare	Biederman et al., 2003
Behavioral phenotype syndromes	0.7%	O'Brien, 2006
(Rare) epilepsy syndromes	0.01–0.4%	Aicardi et al., 2009
PANDAS	Unknown	Swedo et al., 2010
RAD	1%	Sadiq et al., 2012
Total taking overlap into account	7–10%	Gillberg, 1995

Key	ESSENCE	Prevalence
	ADHD	5%
	ODD	4%
	TDs	1%
	RAD	1%
	ASD	1%
	SLI	4-6%
	DCD	5%
	IDD	1.5%
	Epilepsy	0.4%

Figure 3.1.
Overlap of the various syndromes subsumed under the ESSENCE umbrella. Figure by
S. Lundström.

they currently drive development in the whole field of child health, and
all of them have links to one or more of the other conditions/disorders
on the list. Figure 3.1 illustrates—in simplified two-dimensional for-
mat—the complex overlap of the various syndromes subsumed under the
ESSENCE label.

AN EXAMPLE FROM THE FIELD OF SLI

In a recent population study, Miniscalco and colleagues (2006) identified
25 children with SLI at age 2.5 years. They had been screened by child
health nurses and had screened positive (on one or more of the following items: (i) fewer than 25 communicative words, (ii) comprehension
difficulties, (iii) articulation difficulties) *and* been deemed to have some
degree of speech and language impairment after formal testing by a pediatric speech and language therapist (SLT). They were contrasted with 80
children from the general population without SLI and followed as regards
speech and language development for 5 years (seen by an SLT at ages 4,

6, and 7.5 years). When they were 7.5 years old they were, in addition, examined by a neuropsychiatric team, who remained blind to the original assessments. At this age, more than 70% of the children with SLT had ADHD, ASD, IDD, or BIF (or combinations of these). None of them had been suspected of having any of these problems at the original diagnosis of SLI. By age 4 and 6 years, only a small fraction had been recognized to suffer from ADHD or ASD, and an even smaller proportion had received appropriate interventions for such problems.

What can we conclude on the basis of these and similar findings from previous studies? Children with SLI at 2.5 years are a large group—several percent are affected according to U.K. and Swedish studies (Law et al., 2008; Miniscalco et al., 2005). When a child is recognized as having SLI in a child health setting he or she is usually referred for a hearing test and assessment and possibly for speech and language therapy to a pediatric SLT. The results of the study referred to indicate that this might not be appropriate. It would probably be reasonable to characterize the problem signaled by the SLI as belonging to the ESSENCE group and refer the child for multidisciplinary evaluation by a community pediatrician, a psychologist, and an SLT.

AN EXAMPLE FROM THE FIELD OF ASD

Two decades ago, our group demonstrated that autism diagnoses made before age 3 years were relatively stable over time, 75% of patients still meeting the criteria for ASD at follow-up years later (Gillberg et al., 1990). However, in 25% this was not the case, but all the children in this latter group met the criteria for another developmental disorder, such as IDD without ASD, or ADHD. In a new study of more than 300 preschool children with a clinical diagnosis of ASD, the vast majority met the research DSM-IV criteria for autistic disorder, Asperger disorder, or pervasive developmental disorder not otherwise specified at follow-up after 2 years. However, about one in 10 were not diagnosed with ASD but had other developmental disorder diagnoses, such as ADHD, IDD, BIF, SLI, or combinations of these (Fernell et al., 2010). Rates of "comorbid" speech and language problems, ADHD, DCD, gastrointestinal problems, epilepsy, IDD, or BIF in the ASD group varied from about 10% to 60%, but this had not been revealed in connection with the original clinical diagnosis of ASD. The findings provide good support for the notion that these were children suffering from ESSENCE, and, depending on the inclination, interest, and training of the professional first seeing the child because of ESSENCE problems, the child may first have been diagnosed with ADHD, IDD, SLI, or ASD, and any number of the comorbid problems might have been missed.

THE EARLY SYMPTOMS OF ESSENCE

The "typical" symptoms of ESSENCE are listed in Table 3.2. These symptoms should not be seen as "specific" for ESSENCE. Rather, they should be taken as markers for the (very likely) presence of a neurodevelopmental disorder that (very likely) will continue to cause symptoms long after their clinical surfacing in the first few years of life.

TABLE 3.2.
SYMPTOMS (CAUSING MAJOR IMPAIRMENT AND CONCERN FOR 6 MONTHS OR MORE) SIGNALING ESSENCE IN THE FIRST FIVE YEARS OF LIFE

Symptom	Reference
Motor abnormality	Gillberg, 2009
General developmental delay	Gillberg, 2009
Speech and language delay	Law, 2008
Social interaction/communication problems	Wing, 2005
Behavior problems	Hill et al., 2006
Hyperactivity/impulsivity	Biederman et al., 2003
Hypoactivity	Lundervold et al., 2011
Inattention/does not listen	Bishop et al., 1999
Sleep problems	Stores, 2006
Feeding difficulties	Wright et al., 2010

SCOPE OF THE PROBLEM

The estimated prevalence rates of the syndromes subsumed under the ESSENCE acronym are listed in Table 3.1. Most of the disorders listed have been epidemiologically surveyed during the early or middle school ages, and only a few have been the subject of prevalence studies in the preschool years. Even though all of the syndromes are present (and usually symptomatic) from the preschool years, many cases will not have come to the attention of clinicians before school age. Thus, the sum prevalence of about 10% of the general population of children suffering from these syndromes may not reflect how many children come to clinical attention during the preschool period. On the basis of preschool studies of ASD, ODD, and ADHD (Fernell & Gillberg, 2010; Kadesjö et al., 2003), a reasonable estimate would be that about 5% to 7% of children under age 6 years would meet the "criteria" for ESSENCE (i.e., have clinical symptoms of a syndrome and have presented at a clinic with a view to diagnosis and intervention). Boys would be extremely overrepresented in this group, even though they probably wouldn't outnumber girls by more than 2 to 3:1 had parents, teachers, and clinicians been more aware that girls with ASD, ADHD, ODD, and SLI, while meeting the full criteria for these disorders, might have a slightly/clearly different pattern of comorbidity (Kopp et al., 2010; Mahone and Hoffman 2007; Pinkhardt et al., 2009). Girls, as a group, tend to be less violent, less motorically active, more socially adept, and better at using language skills for communication. All of these factors contribute to masking the early symptomatic presentation of disorders such as ASD and ADHD. With better awareness about the presence of such disorders in preschool girls, more and more female cases are likely to come to attention over the next several years.

ADHD (AND ODD AND CONDUCT DISORDER)

ADHD (with or without ODD) is a very common condition, affecting at least 5% of school-age children (Faraone et al., 2003). It is the most common of all the neurodevelopmental disorders/ESSENCE.

In about 60% of the cases identified in the preschool years, ADHD is associated with ODD, which is usually symptomatic by around 3 years of age (Kadesjö et al., 2003). About 10% to 20% of all cases of ADHD (usually recruited from the group of ADHD *plus* ODD) later meet the criteria for conduct disorder, who in turn often meet the full criteria for antisocial personality disorder in adult age. Again, boys are affected much more often than girls, and particularly in the preschool period it is unusual for a girl to be recognized as having the disorder of ADHD (unless it is in the context of having another diagnosis, such as ASD or learning disability).

In about 50% of the cases, ADHD is associated with DCD, and the majority of these patients also have evidence of other learning problems. ODD is quite uncommon in this "ADHD subgroup" (in Scandinavia often referred to as DAMP—i.e., ADHD *plus* DCD). The outcome for the ADHD plus DCD subgroup is also relatively poor in many cases, but this is usually associated with the consequences of academic failure rather than through a more "primary" antisocial pathway.

Many individuals with ADHD have tics and tic disorders, but these are often not specifically or separately diagnosed unless the differential diagnosis or referral question is "? Tourette syndrome."

ADHD, as we shall see, is also associated with a number of other mental health problems, including depression, and anxiety.

It appears that at least half of individuals diagnosed in childhood with ADHD continue to have impairing ADHD in adult life and that the majority have some remaining problems, even if they do not meet the full criteria for "clinical" ADHD (Dopheide & Pliszka, 2009; Rasmussen & Gillberg, 2000). There is evidence that several aspects of the disorder can be positively affected by short- and long-term interventions combining a psychoeducational and pharmacological approach (Ghuman et al., 2008; Vaughan et al., 2009). There are indications that at least when it comes to certain associated conditions (such as ASD), "comorbidity" needs to influence the choice of intervention in important ways to achieve the best possible outcome (Ollendick et al., 2008). Preschool ODD, perhaps the most common of all the associated problems in the field of ADHD, indicates a much increased risk that the child may go on to develop conduct disorder, which in turn is a strong predictor of later antisocial personality disorder.

Recognizing and intervening for ODD in ADHD would probably amelio-rate the prognosis in a number of cases. Similarly, recognizing and inter-vening for DCD in ADHD has the potential of improving outcomes even further. DCD in ADHD is also a strong predictor/marker for associated ASD (Kadesjö & Gillberg, 1999).

ADHD is largely genetic (Curatolo et al., 2009), but a very similar phe-notype can develop after various types of brain damage/environmentally caused brain dysfunction (Strang-Karlsson et al., 2008). The brain devel-ops differently in children with ADHD than in typically developing chil-dren, with loss of the prefrontal component of normal asymmetrical brain development (Shaw et al., 2009). There is also growing evidence that the brain's dopamine-dependent reward system is dysfunctional in ADHD (Volkow et al., 2009). Interestingly, there is now good evidence that ASD and ADHD are clearly related in some families, and that the central ner-vous system connectivity genes involved in ASD may also be relevant for the development of ADHD symptoms (Kopp et al., 2010; Mulligan et al., 2009; Sharp et al., 2009).

ADHD is usually not a discrete disorder. Instead, even in the commu-nity, not just in clinics dealing with severely impaired individuals, "comor-bidity" is the rule (Kadesjö & Gillberg, 2001). ODD, DCD, depression, anxiety, ASD, substance use disorder, and conduct disorder are all rela-tively or very common coexisting disorders. All these "coexisting disor-ders" in ADHD, of course, have an important subgroup of patients within their diagnostic category who have marked attention/impulsivity prob-lems and sometimes meet the full criteria for ADHD.

ASD

ASD is no longer considered a rare condition (Baird et al., 2006); rather, its prevalence during the school years is believed to be slightly higher than 1% of the general population of children. Boys are clearly much more often affected than girls, at least if we are referring to the clinically impair-ing variant of the autism phenotype. Skuse (2009) has argued that the autism phenotype might be equally common in males and females and that other factors are responsible for the large discrepancy in male: female ratios seen in clinical and epidemiological populations. However, others (including Baron-Cohen et al., 2001) have proposed that the autistic phenotype is an expression of the "extreme male brain," which would make the male preponderance in ASD a very real thing and not due to gender roles, comorbidity, or other factors making boys more likely to be diagnosed with the condition.

ASD is a group of multifactorially determined conditions, and there are almost as many different causes as there are cases (Gillberg & Coleman, 2000). The prefrontal, temporal, brainstem, and cerebellar regions of the central nervous system are usually affected. These areas constitute a functional network, "the default network," that appears to be critically differently functioning in ASD (Buckner & Vincent, 2007; Iacoboni, 2006; Monk et al., 2009). ASD with some degree of cognitive impairment is probably associated with life-long disability in the vast majority of cases (e.g., Billstedt et al., 2005), but it is unclear to what extent higher-functioning individuals with ASD (including the group with Asperger syndrome, Table 3.4) continue to show pervasive impairments in adult life (e.g., Cederlund et al., 2010), even though there are indications that persistence of some problems throughout life is more common than not. There is now increasing evidence that early intensive training programs have some lasting beneficial effects on a number of aspects of the disorder, even though the effectiveness of such programmes in daily clinical practice is still a matter of some debate (Fernell et al., 2011)

ASD is almost never an isolated phenomenon (Table 3.3). Coexisting problems and disorders are the rule. These include learning disability (including NVLD), epilepsy, motor control problems, ADHD, depression and anxiety, gastrointestinal problems, and sleep disorders. These problems and disorders are sometimes the reason for referral to a specialist for evaluation. For instance, it is not uncommon for an extremely hyperactive child to be referred for evaluation of ADHD, but the full appraisal, once considered, will reveal that the child's main diagnosis is ASD, and coexisting ADHD may or may not be diagnosed.

TABLE 3.3.

AUTISM SPECTRUM DISORDER CRITERIA ACCORDING TO DSM-5

Autism Spectrum Disorder	
Diagnostic Criteria	**299.00 (F84.0)**

A. Persistent deficits in social communication and social interaction across multiple contexts, as manifested by the following, currently or by history (examples are illustrative, not exhaustive; see text):

    1. Deficits in social-emotional reciprocity, ranging, for example, from abnormal social approach and failure of normal back-and-forth conversation; to reduced sharing of interests, emotions, or affect; to failure to initiate or respond to social interactions.

    2. Deficits in nonverbal communicative behaviors used for social interaction, ranging, for example, from poorly integrated verbal and nonverbal communication; to abnormalities in eye contact and body language or deficits in understanding and use of gestures; to a total lack of facial expressions and nonverbal communication.

    3. Deficits in developing, maintaining, and understanding relationships, ranging, for example, from difficulties adjusting behavior to suit various social contexts; to difficulties in sharing imaginative play or in making friends; to absence of interest in peers.

    Specify current severity:

        Severity is based on social communication impairments and restricted, repetitive patterns of behavior (seeTable 2).

B. Restricted, repetitive patterns of behavior, interests, or activities, as manifested by at least two of the following, currently or by history (examples are illustrative, not exhaustive; see text):

    1. Stereotyped or repetitive motor movements, use of objects, or speech (e.g., simple motor stereotypies, lining up toys or flipping objects, echolalia, idiosyncratic phrases).

    2. Insistence on sameness, inflexible adherence to routines, or ritualized patterns of verbal or nonverbal behavior (e.g., extreme distress at small changes, difficulties with transitions, rigid thinking patterns, greeting rituals, need to take same route or eat same food every day).

    3. Highly restricted, fixated interests that are abnormal in intensity or focus (e.g., strong attachment to or preoccupation with unusual objects, excessively circumscribed or perseverative interests).

    4. Hyper- or hyporeactivity to sensory input of unusual interest in sensory aspects of the environment (e.g., apparent indifference to pain/temperature, adverse response to specific sounds or textures, excessive smelling or touching of objects, visual fascination with lights or movement).

(continued)

TABLE 3.3.
(CONTINUED)

Autism Spectrum Disorder	
Diagnostic Criteria	**299.00 (F84.0)**

Specify current severity:

> **Severity is based on social communication impairments and restricted, repetitive patterns of behavior** (see Table 2).

C. Symptoms must be present in the early developmental period (but may not become fully manifest until social demands exceed limited capacities, or may be masked by learned strategies in later life).

D. Symptoms cause clinically significant impairment in social, occupational, or other important areas of current functioning.

E. These disturbances are not better explained by intellectual disability (intellectual developmental disorder) or global developmental delay. Intellectual disability and autism spectrum disorder frequently co-occur; to make comorbid diagnoses of autism spectrum disorder and intellectual disability, social communication should be below that expected for general developmental level.

Note: Individuals with a well-established DSM-IV diagnosis of autistic disorder, Asperger's disorder, or pervasive developmental disorder not otherwise specified should be given the diagnosis of autism spectrum disorder. Individuals who have marked deficits in social communication, but whose symptoms do not otherwise meet criteria for autism spectrum disorder, should be evaluated for social (pragmatic) communication disorder.

Specify if:

> **With or without accompanying intellectual impairment**
> **With or without accompanying language impairment**
> **Associated with a known medical or genetic condition or environmental factor (Coding note:** Use additional code to identify the associated medical or genetic condition.)
> **Associated with another neurodevelopmental, mental, or behavioral disorder (Coding note:** Use additional code[s] to identify the associated neurodevelopmental, menial, or behavioral disorder[s].)
> **With catatonia** (refer to the criteria for catatonia associated with another mental disorder, pp. 119–120, for definition) **(Coding note:** Use additional code 293.89 [F06.1] catatonia associated with autism spectrum disorder to indicate the presence of the comorbid catatonia.)

IDD, NVLD, AND DYSLEXIA

Learning problems, including intellectual disability (IDD), borderline intellectual functioning, NVLD, and precursors of dyslexia (including phonological awareness problems) are common in the preschool period and affect several percent of both boys and girls. More often than not, such learning problems coexist with other neurodevelopmental/neuropsychiatric disorders, such as ADHD, ASD, and ODD. There is currently a clinical diagnostic substitution trend, at least in the United Kingdom, Scandinavia, and the United States(Bishop et al., 2008; Coo et al., 2008; Fernell & Ek, 2010; Howlin, 2008), leading to fewer children being diagnosed with learning disability and more being labeled as suffering from ASD. The problem with this trend is that the very real learning problems suffered by many individuals with ASD and ADHD may go undiagnosed for long periods of time. In the past, the opposite was often true. NVLD is common in Asperger syndrome (Cederlund and Gillberg 2004; Klin et al., 1995) but is often not recognized and much less diagnosed. This is unhelpful for patients who are clearly impaired by "both conditions." Many individuals with Asperger syndrome—and their parents and teachers—benefit greatly from a better understanding of the particular neuropsychological profile (with its characteristic peaks and troughs) associated with NVLD. The reverse is also true, and Asperger syndrome is often missed by neuropsychologists who specialize in NVLD. Phonological awareness problems, a common precursor of dyslexia, are common in ADHD (with or without associated autistic symptoms) but are often missed once the "overshadowing" diagnosis of ADHD/ASD has been established (Åsberg et al., 2010). Many of these clinical problems, stemming from the over focus on one or other of all the preschool neurodevelopmental disorders, could be avoided if clinicians were more aware of the implications of ESSENCE and had several different diagnoses (and associated/comorbid diagnoses) in mind whenever examining a child presenting with impairing symptoms of ESSENCE.

TABLE 3.4.
ASPERGER SYNDROME BY GILLBERG (IN ACCORDANCE WITH HANS
ASPERGER'S OWN CASE DESCRIPTIONS)

1. **Severe impairment in reciprocal social interaction (at least two of the following)**
   (a) inability to interact with peers
   (b) lack of desire to interact with peers
   (c) lack of appreciation of social cues
   (d) socially and emotionally inappropriate behavior

2. **All-absorbing narrow interest (at least one of the following)**
   (a) exclusion of other activities
   (b) repetitive adherence
   (c) more rote than meaning

3. **Imposition of routines and interests (at least one of the following)**
   (a) on self, in several aspects of life
   (b) on others

4. **Speech and language problems (at least three of the following)**
   (a) delayed development of speech and language
   (b) superficially perfect expressive language
   (c) formal, pedantic language
   (d) odd prosody, peculiar voice characteristics (high pitch, volume unadjusted to situation)
   (e) impairment of comprehension including misinterpretations of literal/ implied meanings

5. **Nonverbal communication problems (at least one of the following)**
   (a) limited use of gestures
   (b) clumsy/gauche body language
   (c) limited facial expression
   (d) inappropriate expression
   (e) peculiar, stiff gaze

6. **Motor clumsiness: poor performance on neurodevelopmental examination (including observed clumsiness)**

Social criterion must always be met. In addition four (three) of the five other criteria must be met for confirmation of diagnosis in males (females).

Criteria by Gillberg and Gillberg (1989) elaborated by Gillberg (1991)

DCD (DEVELOPMENTAL COORDINATION DISORDER)

DCD has recently become the subject of more intense systematic study after having been virtually neglected as an important clinical problem and focus of research. It is quite common, affecting about 5% of all school-age children (Gillberg & Kadesjö, 2003), the majority of whom should be recognizable before age 6 years. However, currently, it is rare for a child to be given this diagnosis before school age. All child psychiatrists should be trained in the field of motor coordination assessment, and pediatricians and other "non-psychiatry" physicians should keep abreast of developments in the field of ADHD and ASD, the two psychiatric disorders that appear to be most commonly associated with DCD. A Swedish population study has suggested that there might be a specific connection between ADHD and ASD, and that it is mediated by DCD (Kadesjö & Gillberg, 1999): children with ADHD who also have DCD (about half the group of all with ADHD) have a very high risk of also having impairing autistic symptomatology, whereas those without DCD have a low risk, and a much higher risk for ODD and conduct problems (Table 3.5).

TICS AND TOURETTE SYNDROME

Tics are extremely common in middle childhood and probably affect at least 15% of all children at some time. Severe, chronic motor and vocal tics (the combination that is referred to as Tourette syndrome) are much less common, probably affecting about 1% of all school-age children (Kadesjö & Gillberg, 2000). Tics fluctuate in intensity and over time, which means that even some severely affected individuals may not actually show any tics during consultation. Tics are rarely diagnosed in the preschool years, but various forerunners of Tourette disorder (such as hyperactivity/impulsivity and a variety of obsessive-compulsive phenomena) are usually present long before the typical, sometimes striking, even dramatic, tics occur or surface at early school age. Tourette disorder

TABLE 3.5.
DEVELOPMENTAL COORDINATION DISORDER CRITERIA ACCORDING
TO DSM-5

Developmental Coordination Disorder	
Diagnostic Criteria	**315.4 (F82)**
A. The acquisition and execution of coordinated motor skills is substantially below that expected given the individual's chronological age and opportunity for skill learning and use. Difficulties are manifested as clumsiness (e.g., dropping or bumping into objects) as well as slowness and inaccuracy of performance of motor skills (e.g., catching an object, using scissors or cutlery, handwriting, riding a bike, or participating in sports).	
B. The motor skills deficit in Criterion A significantly and persistently interferes with activities of daily living appropriate to chronological age (e.g., self-care and self-maintenance) and impacts academic/school productivity, prevocational and vocational activities, leisure, and play.	
C. Onset of symptoms is in the early developmental period.	
D. The motor skills deficits are not better explained by intellectual disability (intellectual developmental disorder) or visual impairment and are not attributable to a neurological condition affecting movement (e.g., cerebral palsy, muscular dystrophy, degenerative disorder).	

Reprinted with permission from the Diagnostic and Statistical Manual of Mental Disorders, Fifth Edition, (Copyright 2013). American Psychiatric Association.

is considered to be a strongly genetic disorder (but more heterogeneous than previously believed) (Keen-Kim & Freimer, 2006; State et al., 2001).

One of the clinically most important aspects of Tourette syndrome (and other severe motor or vocal tic disorders) is its strong association with ADHD and OCD (Debes et al., 2009). Almost all severely handicapped children with Tourette syndrome are affected by either ADHD or OCD or both, and they are usually more impaired by these "comorbid" conditions than by the tic disorder itself (Table 3.6). These associated problems, particularly ADHD (and perhaps particularly extremes of impulsive-hyperactive behaviors), are often apparent during the preschool years, and they, rather than the tics, are what will lead to referral for clinical neurodevelopmental/neuropsychiatric examination.

TABLE 3.6.
TIC DISORDERS CRITERIA ACCORDING TO DSM-5

Tic Disorders	
Diagnostic Criteria	
Note: A tic is a sudden, rapid, recurrent, nonrhythmic motor movement or vocalization.	
Tourette's Disorder	**307.23 (F95.2)**
A. Both multiple motor and one or more vocal tics have been present at some time during the illness, although not necessarily concurrently. B. The tics may wax and wane in frequency but have persisted for more than 1 year since first tic onset. C. Onset is before age 18 years. D. The disturbance is not attributable to the physiological effects of a substance (e.g., cocaine) or another medical condition (e.g., Huntington's disease, postviral encephalitis).	
Persistent (Chronic) Motor or Vocal Tic Disorder	**307.22 (F95.1)**
A. Single or multiple motor or vocal tics have been present during the illness, but not both motor and vocal. B. The tics may wax and wane in frequency but have persisted for more than 1 year since first tic onset. C. Onset is before age 18 years. D. The disturbance is not attributable to the physiological effects of a substance (e.g., cocaine) or another medical condition (e.g., Huntington's disease, postviral encephalitis). E. Criteria have never been met for Tourette's disorder.	
Specify if:	
With motor tics only **With vocal tics only**	
Provisional Tic Disorder	**307.21 (F95.0)**
A. Single or multiple motor and/or vocal tics. B. The tics have been present for less than 1 year since first tic onset. C. Onset is before age 18 years. D. The disturbance is not attributable to the physiological effects of a substance (e.g., cocaine) or another medical condition (e.g., Huntington's disease, postviral encephalitis). E. Criteria have never been met for Tourette's disorder or persistent (chronic) motor or vocal tic disorder.	

BIPOLAR DISORDER

Pediatric bipolar disorder is still a somewhat controversial diagnosis (Biederman et al., 1989). However, it is becoming increasingly recognized that bipolar disorder can present with symptoms in the preschool years. Children with "ADHD" and/or depression who have a family history of bipolar disorder may actually be presenting with signs and symptoms of a bipolar disorder (Chang, 2008). Extremes of irritability, mood swings, and even classic manic symptoms may appear in the first several years of life and signal the possibility of an underlying bipolar disorder. ADHD and ASD can both occur in conjunction with bipolar disorder (and can probably overshadow the affective disorder). Longitudinal systematic study of large groups of children with ESSENCE will help clarify the prevalence and importance of pediatric bipolar disorder (Table 3.7).

BEHAVIORAL PHENOTYPE SYNDROMES

More than 1.0% of all preschool children may be affected by one (or more) of the "rare disorders," also referred to as behavioral phenotype syndromes (Gillberg, 2010). Examples of such disorders are the fragile X syndrome, 22q11deletion syndrome, 22q13 syndrome, neurofibromatosis, tuberous sclerosis, and Smith-Lemli-Opitz syndrome. Each of these disorders is really "rare" (occurring usually in fewer than 1 in 2,000 children), but given that there are hundreds of them, taken as a group they are actually quite common. The majority of these syndromes have a large subgroup—usually the majority—with some degree of cognitive impairment, although many affected individuals do not have learning disability, and some have a high IQ (e.g., most individuals with Marfan syndrome and about half the group with 22q11deletion syndrome). Large subgroups of individuals within each category of the rare disorders in addition have ASD or ADHD or both, and other individuals may have other neuropsychiatric/neurodevelopmental problems that are symptomatic from a very young age (Gillberg, I. C., et al., 1994; Hagerman et al., 2009; Niklasson

TABLE 3.7.
BIPOLAR I & BIPOLAR II DISORDER CRITERIA ACCORDING TO DSM-5

Bipolar I Disorder
Diagnostic Criteria
For a diagnosis of bipolar I disorder, it is necessary to meet the following criteria for a manic episode. The manic episode may have been preceded by and may be followed by hypomanic or major depressive episodes. **Manic Episode** A. A distinct period of abnormally and persistently elevated, expansive, or irritable mood and abnormally and persistently increased goal-directed activity or energy, lasting at least 1 week and present most of the day, nearly every day (or any duration if hospitalization is necessary). B. During the period of mood disturbance and increased energy or activity, three (or more) of the following symptoms (four if the mood is only irritable) are present to a significant degree and represent a noticeable change from usual behavior: 1. Inflated self-esteem or grandiosity. 2. Decreased need for sleep (e.g., feels rested after only 3 hours of sleep). 3. More talkative than usual or pressure to keep talking. 4. Flight of ideas or subjective experience that thoughts are racing. 5. Distractibility (i.e., attention too easily drawn to unimportant or irrelevant external stimuli), as reported or observed. 6. Increase in goal-directed activity (either socially, at work or school, or sexually) or psychomotor agitation (i.e., purposeless non-goal-directed activity). 7. Excessive involvement in activities that have a high potential for painful consequences (e.g., engaging in unrestrained buying sprees, sexual indiscretions, or foolish business investments). C. The mood disturbance is sufficiently severe to cause marked impairment in social or occupational functioning or to necessitate hospitalization to prevent harm to self or others, or there are psychotic features. D. The episode is not attributable to the physiological effects of a substance (e.g., a drug of abuse, a medication, other treatment) or to another medical condition.

TABLE 3.7.
(CONTINUED)

Note: A full manic episode that emerges during antidepressant treatment (e.g., medication, electroconvulsive therapy) but persists at a fully syndromal level beyond the physiological effect of that treatment is sufficient evidence for a manic episode and, therefore, a bipolar I diagnosis. **Note:** Criteria A–D constitute a manic episode. At least one lifetime manic episode is required for the diagnosis of bipolar I disorder.
Hypomanic Episode
A. A distinct period of abnormally and persistently elevated, expansive, or irritable mood and abnormally and persistently increased activity or energy, lasting at least 4 consecutive days and present most of the day, nearly every day. B. During the period of mood disturbance and increased energy and activity, three (or more) of the following symptoms (four if the mood is only irritable) have persisted, represent a noticeable change from usual behavior, and have been present to a significant degree: 1. Inflated self-esteem or grandiosity. 2. Decreased need for sleep (e.g., feels rested after only 3 hours of sleep). 3. More talkative than usual or pressure to keep talking. 4. Flight of ideas or subjective experience that thoughts are racing. 5. Distractibility (i.e., attention too easily drawn to unimportant or irrelevant external stimuli), as reported or observed. 6. Increase in goal-directed activity (either socially, at work or school, or sexually) or psychomotor agitation. 7. Excessive involvement in activities that have a high potential for painful consequences (e.g., engaging in unrestrained buying sprees, sexual indiscretions, or foolish business investments). C. The episode is associated with an unequivocal change in functioning that is uncharacteristic of the individual when not symptomatic. D. The disturbance in mood and the change in functioning are observable by others. E. The episode is not severe enough to cause marked impairment in social or occupational functioning or to necessitate hospitalization. If there are psychotic features, the episode is, by definition, manic.

(continued)

TABLE 3.7.
(CONTINUED)

F. The episode is not attributable to the physiological effects of a substance
   (e.g., a drug of abuse, a medication, other treatment).
Note: A full hypomanic episode that emerges during antidepressant treatment
(e.g., medication, electroconvulsive therapy) but persists at a fully syndromal
level beyond the physiological effect of that treatment is sufficient evidence for
a hypomanic episode diagnosis. However, caution is indicated so that one or
two symptoms (particularly increased irritability, edginess, or agitation following
antidepressant use) are not taken as sufficient for diagnosis of a hypomanic
episode, nor necessarily indicative of a bipolar diathesis.
Note: Criteria A–F constitute a hypomanic episode. Hypomanic episodes are
common in bipolar I disorder but are not required for the diagnosis of bipolar
I disorder.

Major Depressive Episode

A. Five (or more) of the following symptoms have been present during the same
   2-week period and represent a change from previous functioning; at least
   one of the symptoms is either (1) depressed mood or (2) loss of interest or
   pleasure.
Note: Do not include symptoms that are clearly attributable to another medical
condition.
   1. Depressed mood most of the day, nearly every day, as indicated by either
      subjective report (e.g., feels sad, empty, or hopeless) or observation made
      by others (e.g., appears tearful). (**Note:** In children and adolescents, can
      be irritable mood.)
   2. Markedly diminished interest or pleasure in all, or almost all, activities
      most of the day, nearly every day (as indicated by either subjective
      account or observation).
   3. Significant weight loss when not dieting or weight gain (e.g., a change
      of more than 5% of body weight in a month), or decrease or increase
      in appetite nearly every day. (**Note:** In children, consider failure to make
      expected weight gain.)
   4. Insomnia or hypersomnia nearly every day.
   5. Psychomotor agitation or retardation nearly every day (observable by
      others; not merely subjective feelings of restlessness or being slowed
      down).

TABLE 3.7.
(CONTINUED)

> 6. Fatigue or loss of energy nearly every day.
>
> 7. Feelings of worthlessness or excessive or inappropriate guilt (which may be delusional) nearly every day (not merely self-reproach or guilt about being sick).
>
> 8. Diminished ability to think or concentrate, or indecisiveness, nearly every day (either by subjective account or as observed by others).
>
> 9. Recurrent thoughts of death (not just fear of dying), recurrent suicidal ideation without a specific plan, or a suicide attempt or a specific plan for committing suicide.
>
> B. The symptoms cause clinically significant distress or impairment in social, occupational, or other important areas of functioning.
>
> C. The episode is not attributable to the physiological effects of a substance or another medical condition.
>
> **Note:** Criteria A–C constitute a major depressive episode. Major depressive episodes are common in bipolar I disorder but are not required for the diagnosis of bipolar I disorder.
>
> **Note:** Responses to a significant loss (e.g., bereavement, financial ruin, losses from a natural disaster, a serious medical Illness or disability) may include the feelings of intense sadness, rumination about the loss, insomnia, poor appetite, and weight loss noted in Criterion A, which may resemble a depressive episode. Although such symptoms may be understandable or considered appropriate to the loss, the presence of a major depressive episode in addition to the normal response to a significant loss should also be carefully considered. This decision inevitably requires the exercise of clinical judgment based on the individual's history and the cultural norms for the expression of distress in the context of loss.[1]

---

[1] In distinguishing grief from a major depressive episode (MDE), it is useful to consider that in grief the predominant affect is feelings of emptiness and loss, while in MDE it is persistent depressed mood and the inability to anticipate happiness or pleasure. The dysphoria in grief is likely to decrease in intensity over days to weeks and occurs in waves, the so-called pangs of grief. These waves tend to be associated with thoughts or reminders of the deceased. The depressed mood of a MDE is more persistent and not tied to specific thoughts or preoccupations. The pain of grief may be accompanied by positive emotions and humor that are uncharacteristic of the

(continued)

TABLE 3.7.
(CONTINUED)

Bipolar I Disorder
A. Criteria have been met for at least one manic episode (Criteria A–D under "Manic Episode" above).
B. The occurrence of the manic and major depressive episode(s) is not better explained by schizoaffective disorder, schizophrenia, schizophreniform disorder, delusional disorder, or other specified or unspecified schizophrenia spectrum and other psychotic disorder.

Coding and Recording Procedures

The diagnostic code for bipolar I disorder is based on type of current or most recent episode and its status with respect to current severity, presence of psychotic features, and remission status. Current severity and psychotic features are only indicated if full criteria are currently met for a manic or major depressive episode. Remission specifiers are only indicated if the full criteria are not currently met for a manic, hypomanic, or major depressive episode. Codes are as follows:

Bipolar I disorder	Current or most recent episode manic	Current or most recent episode hypomanic*	Current or most recent episode depressed	Current or most recent episode unspecified**
Mild	296.41 (F31.11)	NA	296.51 (F31.31)	NA
Moderate	296.42 (F31.12)	NA	296.52 (F31.32)	NA
Severe	296.43 (F31.13)	NA	296.53 (F31.4)	NA

pervasive unhappiness and misery characteristic of a major depressive episode. The thought content associated with grief generally features a preoccupation with thoughts and memories of the deceased, rather than the self-critical or pessimistic ruminations seen in a MDE. In grief, self-esteem is generally preserved, whereas in a MDE, feelings of worthlessness and self-loathing are common. If self-derogatory ideation is present in grief, it typically involves perceived failings vis-à-vis the deceased (e.g., not visiting frequently enough, not telling the deceased how much he or she was loved). If a bereaved individual thinks about death and dying, such thoughts are generally focused on the deceased and possibly about "joining" the deceased, whereas in a major depressive episode such thoughts are focused on ending one's own life because of feeling worthless, undeserving of life, or unable to cope with the pain of depression.

TABLE 3.7.
(CONTINUED)

With psychotic features***	296.44 (F31.2)	NA	296.54 (F31.5)	NA
In partial remission	296.45 (F31.73)	296.45 (F31.73)	296.55 (F31.75)	NA
In full remission	296.46 (F31.74)	296.46 (F31.74)	296.56 (F31.76)	NA
Unspecified	296.40 (F31.9)	296.40 (F31.9)	296.50 (F31.9)	NA

*Severity and psychotic specifiers do not apply; code 296.40 (F31.0) for cases not in remission.
**Severity, psychotic, and remission specifiers do not apply. Code 296.7 (F31.9).
***If psychotic features are present, code the "with psychotic features" specifier irrespective of episode severity.

In recording the name of a diagnosis, terms should be listed in the following order: bipolar I disorder, type of current or most recent episode, severity/psychotic/remission specifiers, followed by as many specifiers without codes as apply to the current or most recent episode.

Specify:

With anxious distress

With mixed features

With rapid cycling

With melancholic features

With atypical features

With mood-congruent psychotic features

With mood-incongruent psychotic features

With catatonia. Coding note: Use additional code 293.89 (F06.1).

With peripartum onset

With seasonal pattern

Bipolar II Disorder

Diagnostic Criteria	296.89 (F31.81)

For a diagnosis of bipolar II disorder, it is necessary to meet the following criteria for a current or past hypomanic episode *and* the following criteria for a current or past major depressive episode:

(continued)

TABLE 3.7.
(CONTINUED)

Hypomanic Episode

A. A distinct period of abnormally and persistently elevated, expansive, or irritable mood and abnormally and persistently increased activity or energy, lasting at least 4 consecutive days and present most of the day, nearly every day.

B. During the period of mood disturbance and increased energy and activity, three (or more) of the following symptoms have persisted (four if the mood is only irritable), represent a noticeable change from usual behavior, and have been present to a significant degree:
1. Inflated self-esteem or grandiosity.
2. Decreased need for sleep (e.g., feels rested after only 3 hours of sleep).
3. More talkative than usual or pressure to keep talking.
4. Flight of ideas or subjective experience that thoughts are racing.
5. Distractibility (i.e., attention too easily drawn to unimportant or irrelevant external stimuli), as reported or observed.
6. Increase in goal-directed activity (either socially, at work or school, or sexually) or psychomotor agitation.
7. Excessive involvement in activities that have a high potential for painful consequences (e.g., engaging in unrestrained buying sprees, sexual indiscretions, or foolish business investments).

C. The episode is associated with an unequivocal change in functioning that is uncharacteristic of the individual when not symptomatic.

D. The disturbance in mood and the change in functioning are observable by others.

E. The episode is not severe enough to cause marked impairment in social or occupational functioning or to necessitate hospitalization. If there are psychotic features, the episode is, by definition, manic.

F. The episode is not attributable to the physiological effects of a substance (e.g., a drug of abuse, a medication or other treatment).

Note: A full hypomanic episode that emerges during antidepressant treatment (e.g., medication, electroconvuisive therapy) but persists at a fully syndromal level beyond the physiological effect of that treatment is sufficient evidence for a hypomanic episode diagnosis. However, caution is indicated so that one or two symptoms (particularly increased irritability, edginess, or agitation following antidepressant use) are not taken as sufficient for diagnosis of a hypomanic episode, nor necessarily indicative of a bipolar diathesis.

TABLE 3.7.
(CONTINUED)

Major Depressive Episode

A. Five (or more) of the following symptoms have been present during the same 2-week period and represent a change from previous functioning; at least one of the symptoms is either (1) depressed mood or (2) loss of interest or pleasure.

Note: Do not include symptoms that are clearly attributable to a medical condition.

  1. Depressed mood most of the day, nearly every day, as indicated by either subjective report (e.g., feels sad, empty, or hopeless) or observation made by others (e.g., appears tearful). (**Note:** In children and adolescents, can be irritable mood.)
  2. Markedly diminished interest or pleasure in all, or almost all, activities most of the day, nearly every day (as indicated by either subjective account or observation).
  3. Significant weight loss when not dieting or weight gain (e.g., a change of more than 5% of body weight in a month), or decrease or increase in appetite nearly every day. (**Note:** In children, consider failure to make expected weight gain.)
  4. Insomnia or hypersomnia nearly every day.
  5. Psychomotor agitation or retardation nearly every day (observable by others; not merely subjective feelings of restlessness or being slowed down).
  6. Fatigue or loss of energy nearly every day.
  7. Feelings of worthlessness or excessive or inappropriate guilt (which may be delusional) nearly every day (not merely self-reproach or guilt about being sick).
  8. Diminished ability to think or concentrate, or indecisiveness, nearly every day (either by subjective account or as observed by others).
  9. Recurrent thoughts of death (not just fear of dying), recurrent suicidal ideation without a specific plan, a suicide attempt, or a specific plan for committing suicide.

B. The symptoms cause clinically significant distress or impairment in social, occupational, or other important areas of functioning.

C. The episode is not attributable to the physiological effects of a substance or another medical condition.

(continued)

TABLE 3.7.
(CONTINUED)

Note: Criteria A–C above constitute a major depressive episode.

Note: Responses to a significant loss (e.g., bereavement, financial ruin, losses from a natural disaster, a serious medical illness or disability) may include the feelings of intense sadness, rumination about the loss, insomnia, poor appetite, and weight loss noted in Criterion A, which may resemble a depressive episode. Although such symptoms may be understandable or considered appropriate to the loss, the presence of a major depressive episode in addition to the normal response to a significant loss should be carefully considered. This decision inevitably requires the exercise of clinical judgment based on the individual's history and the cultural norms for the expression of distress in the context of loss.[1]

Bipolar II Disorder

A. Criteria have been met for at least one hypomanic episode (Criteria A–F under "Hypomanic Episode" above) and at least one major depressive episode (Criteria A–C under "Major Depressive Episode" above).

B. There has never been a manic episode.

C. The occurrence of the hypomanic episode(s) and major depressive episode(s) is not better explained by schizoaffective disorder, schizophrenia, schizophreniform disorder, delusional disorder, or other specified or unspecified schizophrenia spectrum and other psychotic disorder.

---

1. In distinguishing grief from a major depressive episode (MDE), it is useful to consider that in grief the predominant affect is feelings of emptiness and loss, while in a MDE it is persistent depressed mood and the inability to anticipate happiness or pleasure. The dysphoria in grief is likely to decrease in intensity over days to weeks and occurs in waves, the so-called pangs of grief. These waves tend to be associated with thoughts or reminders of the deceased. The depressed mood of a MDE is more persistent and not tied to specific thoughts or preoccupations. The pain of grief may be accompanied by positive emotions and humor that are uncharacteristic of the pervasive unhappiness and misery characteristic of a MDE. The thought content associated with grief generally features a preoccupation with thoughts and memories of the deceased, rather than the self-critical or pessimistic ruminations seen in a MDE. In grief, self-esteem is generally preserved, whereas in a MDE feelings of worthlessness and self-loathing are common. If self-derogatory ideation is present in grief, it typically involves perceived failings vis-à-vis the deceased (e.g., not visiting frequently enough, not telling the deceased how much he or she was loved). If a bereaved individual thinks about death and dying, such thoughts are generally focused on the deceased and possibly about "joining" the deceased, whereas in a MDE such thoughts are focused on ending one's own life because of feeling worthless, undeserving of life, or unable to cope with the pain of depression.

TABLE 3.7.
(CONTINUED)

D. The symptoms of depression or the unpredictability caused by frequent
alternation between periods of depression and hypomania causes clinically
significant distress or impairment in social, occupational, or other important
areas of functioning.

Coding and Recording Procedures

Bipolar II disorder has one diagnostic code: 296.89 (F31.81). Its status with
respect to current severity, presence of psychotic features, course, and other
specifiers cannot be coded but should be indicated in writing (e.g., 296.89
[F31.81] bipolar II disorder, current episode depressed, moderate severity,
with mixed features; 296.89 [F31.81] bipolar II disorder, most recent episode
depressed, in partial remission).

Specify current or most recent episode:

Hypomanic

Depressed

Specify if:

  With anxious distress

  With mixed features

  With rapid cycling

  With mood-congruent psychotic features

  With mood-incongruent psychotic features

  With catatonia. Coding note: Use additional code 293.89 (F06.1).

  With peripartum onset

  With seasonal pattern: Applies only to the pattern of major depressive
  episodes.

Specify course if full criteria for a mood episode are not currently met:

  In partial remission

  In full remission

Specify severity if full criteria for a mood episode are currently met:

  Mild

  Moderate

Severe

---

et al., 2009; Sikora et al., 2006). Indeed, it is very common for such problems to be the original reason for referral. In our center we see quite a number of cases each year in which the behavioral phenotype syndrome (and the genetic abnormality usually underlying it) has been missed.

RARE EPILEPSY SYNDROMES AND FEBRILE SEIZURES

Landau-Kleffner syndrome or "verbal auditory agnosia with seizures" is a relatively rare syndrome that often presents in the preschool years and that is sometimes "misdiagnosed" as ASD, ADHD, or both. Children with Landau-Kleffner syndrome very often meet the criteria for one or both of these types of conditions, but the underlying epileptic syndrome must not remain undiagnosed. Pulsed steroids and in certain cases surgical treatments may be indicated (Cross & Neville, 2009). The overlap with the syndrome referred to as continuous spike wave activity during slow-wave sleep (CSWS) is considerable, and it is probably more a matter of the child's age than of any intrinsic difference between Landau-Kleffner syndrome (preschool children) and CSWS (older children) which of the named conditions gets a label in the individual case. CSWS is probably a much under diagnosed condition that can sometimes underlie a relatively acute onset of a variety of neuropsychiatric symptoms—including ADHD, tic disorders, and OCD—and can probably be both missed and over diagnosed in cases presenting with the PANDAS phenotype (see below).

Infantile spasms (Saemundsen et al., 2008) and Dravet syndrome with SCN1A mutations (Arzimanoglou, 2009) carry high risks of intellectual disability, ASD, and ADHD. It is important that such additional diagnoses are not overlooked in the follow-up of preschool children with these rare epilepsy syndromes, given that clinical experience suggests beneficial effects of ASD and ADHD interventions even in the presence of the severe underlying seizure disorder. Other rare epilepsy syndromes with onset in the preschool period are usually of such devastating character that making additional diagnoses of neuropsychiatric disorders such as

ASD and ADHD is often not discussed or indeed relevant. However, just occasionally, epilepsies of the Lennox-Gastaut type (and other, even rarer conditions) can be sufficiently well controlled and ASD- or ADHD-type problems so pronounced that the issue of ESSENCE might be raised. In such instances it would not be appropriate to conclude that given the nature and severity of the epilepsy syndrome, an additional diagnosis of ASD, ADHD, or another ESSENCE behavior disorder would make little difference. There is sufficient anecdotal support for the notion that even in cases considered "hopeless," interventions targeting ASD and/or ADHD may drastically improve quality of life for affected families.

PANDAS (PEDIATRIC AUTOIMMUNE NEUROPSYCHIATRIC DISORDERS ASSOCIATED WITH *STREPTOCOCCAL* INFECTION)

The term PANDAS was introduced by Swedo to describe a subset of child-hood obsessive-compulsive disorders (OCD) and tic disorders (often with associated symptoms from other categories of ESSENCE) triggered by group-A beta-hemolytic *Streptococcus pyogenes* infection (Swedo et al., 1998). More recently, the acronym PANS (pediatric acute-onset neuro-psychiatric syndrome) has been introduced to account for cases with sim-ilar acute-onset symptomatology but without a proven link specifically to streptococcal infection. Case reports and case series have documented that PANDAS/PANS can present with a wide variety of ESSENCE symptoms, not just OCD and tics, but also ADHD, manic and bipolar symptoms, DCD (specifically acute-onset handwriting difficulties), language regres-sion (and other, usually transient, regressive symptoms), and intrusive thoughts reminiscent of schizophrenia/psychosis. Urinary urgency with an OCD-type quality and acute onset usually combined with separation anxiety should alert the clinician to the possibility of PANDAS/PANS.

Similar to adult OCD, PANDAS is suggested to be associated with basal ganglia dysfunction (Moretti et al., 2008). The symptoms overlap with those of Sydenham chorea. Other putative pathogenetic mechanisms of

PANDAS include molecular mimicry and autoimmune-mediated altered neuronal signaling, involving calcium-calmodulin dependent protein (CaM) kinase II activity. Nonetheless, the contrasting results from numerous studies provide no consensus on whether PANDAS should be considered as a specific nosological entity or simply a useful clinical research framework.

It is still unclear to what extent PANS responds to a variety of treatments, including antibiotics, steroids, or immunoglobulin therapies. A number of case studies suggest that such (early) interventions could be of considerable positive effect. The relative dearth of research into the fascinating area of autoimmunity and early-onset neurodevelopmental disorders is surprising, given the strong upsurge in interest demonstrated already more than a decade ago (Dale & Heyman, 2002).

RAD (REACTIVE ATTACHMENT DISORDER)

There is emerging evidence that RAD as defined under the DSM-IV-TR/DSM-5 exists as a relatively distinct problem (Minnis et al., 2009). It can be recognized in the preschool years (Zeanah et al., 2003) and separated from—although symptomatically overlapping with—ADHD during the early school years (Minnis et al., 2009). It also is associated with severe pragmatic language problems that are not explained by the occasional co-occurrence with ASD (Sadiq et al., 2012). It is of considerable interest that a large subgroup of children meeting symptomatic criteria for RAD have not been severely abused or deprived in early childhood (Minnis et al., 2009). A brief screen for the disorder is available for school-age children (Minnis et al., 2002), but there is a need for development of more refined screening and diagnostic tools for preschoolers. The disorder should be considered in all children who have suffered severe maltreatment or deprivation in the early years, and perhaps also in all children with any kind of impairing ESSENCE symptom who show the possibly discriminating feature of overfriendliness, indeed sometimes even cuddliness, with strangers (Minnis et al., 2009).

OVERLAP, COEXISTENCE, AND "COMORBIDITY"

The word "comorbidity" is inadequate when it comes to describing and delineating the reality and meaning of the co-occurrence of phenomena, problems, symptoms, syndromes and disorders, and diseases in the clinical and research fields of ESSENCE. Most clinicians and researchers attach different meanings to the word "comorbidity"(Caron & Rutter, 1991). Using the word in a literal sense, one would assume that a person diagnosed with "comorbid" ASD and ADHD would have two different morbid ("disease") conditions. These morbid conditions could have different etiologies, the same etiology, or no known etiology ("idiopathic"). In actual fact, when we talk about comorbidity, what we are usually referring to is "coexistence," "association," "overlap," "additional problems" or suchlike. When the word "comorbidity" has been used here (usually within quotes), it has been "in that sense."

The syndromes subsumed under the ESSENCE label constitute collections of symptoms—sometimes, but certainly not always, operationalized under rigidly structured algorithms—that, at the current state of our knowledge, appear to delineate clinically meaningful conditions. However, as our knowledge base increases, so the algorithm barriers for making the specific diagnoses will need to be reviewed and, quite often, changed. This has happened over the past 30 years in ASD and ADHD. The DSM-5 introduces another, probably major, change in how these categories are conceptualized, operationalized, algorithmized, and diagnosed. There is growing realization that (a) most so-called syndromes, including ADHD, DCD, IDD, and ASD, are, at least to some extent, partly arbitrary endpoints or cutoff points on normal distribution curves, and depending on where you draw the line, you may be referring to autistic disorder or Asperger syndrome; (b) most syndromes comprise a mixture of symptom collections from endpoints or cutoff points of different normal distribution curves, so that, at intersections, some individuals affected will meet the criteria for ASD, others for ASD with ADHD, and others still for ADHD "only"; (c) most syndromes can be "mimicked by" (or may have actually be modeled around) more circumscribed brain disorders (genetic or environmental) or diffuse or unspecific/specific brain injury/ dysfunction (temporary or chronic) caused by a variety of factors, including the effects of myelin disorder after extreme prematurity, periventricular bleeding after perinatal asphyxia, thalidomide—or extremes of alcohol—exposure in fetal life, and exposure to products included in diets currently considered to be "normal," or at least not harmful. Against this background, it should come as no surprise that the introduction of the term ESSENCE, as suggested by the definition of the acronym, is nothing but an attempt to acknowledge this state of affairs, and the fact that we need to implement this approach to thinking about the problems in the whole wide field of child health and development services.

THE IMPLICATIONS OF ESSENCE

In summary, the reasons why a term such as ESSENCE is needed at this point in time in child psychiatry, developmental medicine, and child neurology, are as follows:

ESSENCE is a new "label" but *not* a new way of thinking about
   early-onset problems that continue to affect children's development
   long after the preschool period.
ESSENCE is intended to query the current trend toward
   compartmentalizing syndromes in child and adolescent
   psychiatry and developmental medicine to the extent that
   "things" such as ADHD, DCD, and ASD are considered
   "boxes" that are exclusive and always separable from
   each other.
ESSENCE draws attention to the fact that there is no simple solution
   to diagnosis in young children who present with symptoms
   indicating ESSENCE. All children presenting with an ESSENCE
   problem need a holistic approach and need to be considered from
   the point of view of "multiproblems" and the possible need for
   multidisciplinary assessment and intervention.

The overlap of problems encountered in the field of ESSENCE indicates that ADHD, DCD, ASD, and so forth are not discrete disorders or syndromes. They share underlying genetic and epigenetically driven brain dysfunctions/neurodevelopmental problems that reflect circuitry breakdown, network dysfunctions, and decreased/aberrant/increased connectivity or, indeed, in some cases, "normal" brain function variants. Therefore, it would be inappropriate to diagnose one problem and not consider the implications of the other(s). The trend toward delivering services and clinics specifically for ADHD, Tourette syndrome, or ASD does not appear to be helpful. In the future, as we learn more about the extent of normality, and about the fact that we are all different, there may not be a need for lumping together diagnoses (such as ESSENCE) but for specific diagnosis of genetic and environmental contributors to the problems encountered in each individual case.

All of the above would appear to combine to suggest the obvious solution. there is a need for child ESSENCE centers (rather than separate behavioral pediatrics, child psychiatry, child neurology, SLT services, special education units, ADHD, Tourette, ASD, or affective disorder centers) to be organized for all preschool and school-age children, catering to the diagnostic medical assessment, intervention planning, and follow-up requirements that are clearly warranted for the vast majority of children presenting with a major ESSENCE symptom. There is abundant evidence that major problems in at least one ESSENCE domain before age 5 years signal major problems in the same or overlapping domains several years later. There is no time to "sit down and wait"; something needs to be done, and that something is unlikely to be "just" in the area of hyperactivity and inattention, speech and language, "just" in the area of social communication, or "just" in special education.

The development of problems in ESSENCE from pregnancy through the early years and adolescence into adult life is depicted in Figure 3.2.

Progress in medical research often leads to refinement of diagnostic criteria and more precise methods of subgrouping according to etiology, with consequences for intervention. Superficially, this much-accepted view of evidence-based medicine could be seen as support for a "splitter"

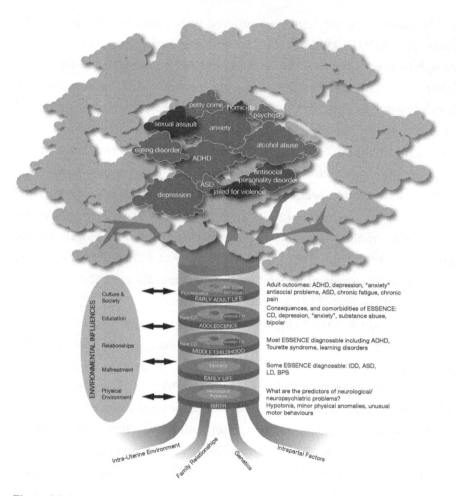

Figure 3.2.
ESSENCE through the lifespan. Graphics prepared by S. Graham.

approach to medical progress. The introduction of the ESSENCE label
could, therefore, be taken by some to signal a step back in development in
child psychiatry, child neurology, and pediatrics, given its implicit support
for a "lumper" view. However, lumping of ESSENCE will be meaningful
only if clinicians and researchers *start* by approaching the area of early
child developmental problems by accepting that splitting in a state-of-
the-art way (making detailed and individualized diagnosis and intervention plans) will be possible only if there is anything to start splitting from

(i.e., from a "lumped" group of cases). Also, if splitting occurs already in the mind of the original clinician/referring person (i.e., hyperactivity and behavior problems are seen as the domain of the ADHD specialist, delayed language is seen as the "property" of the SLT, social interaction problems are seen as the "remit" of the "autism center," and delayed overall development with behavior problems is seen as the "business of the learning disability psychiatrist"), this would lead to inadvertent delay in recognizing that the child with ESSENCE very likely will have more than one problem (i.e., ADHD with DCD, ASD with ADHD *and* epilepsy, ADHD with Tourette syndrome, OCD, *and* RAD, etc.).

In summary, the introduction of the ESSENCE mode of thinking about problems to do with deviations from normal child development should not be taken as support for lumping rather than splitting, but for the order in which these two aspects of diagnosis are approached.

REFERENCES

Aicardi, J., Bax, M., & Gillberg, C. (Eds.) (2009). *Diseases of the nervous system in childhood* (3rd ed.). London: Mac Keith Press.

Arzimanoglou, A. (2009). Dravet syndrome: from electroclinical characteristics to molecular biology. *Epilepsia, 50*, Suppl 8, 3–9.

Åsberg, J., Kopp, S., Berg-Kelly, K., & Gillberg, C. (2010). Reading comprehension, word decoding and spelling in girls with autism spectrum disorders (ASD) or attention-deficit/hyperactivity disorder (AD/HD): performance and predictors. *International Journal of Language & Communication Disorders, 45*, 61–71.

Baird, G., Simonoff, E., Pickles, A., Chandler, S., Loucas, T., Meldrumm, D., et al. (2006). Prevalence of disorders of the autism spectrum in a population cohort of children in South Thames: the Special Needs and Autism Project (SNAP). *Lancet, 368*, 210–215.

Baron-Cohen, S., Wheelwright, S., Skinner, R., Martin, J., & Clubley, E. (2001). The autism-spectrum quotient (AQ): evidence from Asperger syndrome/high-functioning autism, males and females, scientists and mathematicians. *Journal of Autism and Developmental Disorders, 31*, 5–17. Erratum in: *Journal of Autism and Developmental Disorders, 31*, 603.

Biederman, J., Mick, E., Faraone, S.V., Spencer, T., Wilens, T.E., & Wozniak, J. (2003). Current concepts in the validity, diagnosis and treatment of paediatric bipolar disorder. *International Journal of Neuropsychopharmacology, 6*, 293–300.

Biederman, J., Baldessarini, R.J., Wright, V., Knee, D., Harmatz, J.S., & Goldblatt, A. (1989). A double-blind placebo controlled study of desipramine in the treatment ADD: II. Serum drug levels and cardiovascular findings. *Journal of the American Academy of Child and Adolescent Psychiatry, 28,* 903–911.

Billstedt, E., Gillberg, I.C., & Gillberg, C. (2005). Autism after adolescence: population-based 13–22-year follow-up study of 120 individuals with autism diagnosed in childhood. *Journal of Autism and Developmental Disorders, 35,* 351–360.

Bishop, D.V., Bishop, S.J., Bright, P., James, C., Delaney, T., & Tallal, P. (1999). Different origin of auditory and phonological processing problems in children with language impairment: evidence from a twin study. *Journal of Speech, Language, and Hearing Research, 42,* 155–168.

Bishop, D.V., Whitehouse, A.J., Watt, H.J., & Line, E.A. (2008). Autism and diagnostic substitution: evidence from a study of adults with a history of developmental language disorder. *Developmental Medicine and Child Neurology, 50,* 341–345.

Buckner, R.L., & Vincent, J.L. (2007). Unrest at rest: default activity and spontaneous network correlations. *NeuroImage, 37,* 1091–1096.

Caron, C., & Rutter, M. (1991). Comorbidity in child psychopathology: concepts, issues and research strategies. *Journal of Child Psychology and Psychiatry, 32,* 1063–1080.

Cederlund, M., & Gillberg, C. (2004). One hundred males with Asperger syndrome: a clinical study of background and associated factors. *Developmental Medicine and Child Neurology, 46,* 652–660.

Cederlund, M., Hagberg, B., & Gillberg, C. (2010). Asperger syndrome in adolescent and young adult males. Interview, self- and parent assessment of social, emotional and cognitive problems. *Research in Developmental Disabilities, 31,* 287–298.

Chang, K.D. (2008). The use of atypical antipsychotics in pediatric bipolar disorder. *Journal of Clinical Psychiatry, 69,* Suppl 4, 4–8.

Coleman, M., & Gillberg, C. (2012). *The autisms* (4th ed.). New York: Oxford University Press.

Comings, D.E. (1990). *Tourette syndrome and human behavior* (1st ed.). Duarte: Hope Press.

Constantino, J.N., Lavesser, P.D., Zhang, Y., Abbacchi, A.M., Gray, T., & Todd, R.D. (2007). Rapid quantitative assessment of autistic social impairment by classroom teachers. *Journal of American Academy of Child and Adolescent Psychiatry, 46,* 1668–1676.

Coo, H., Ouellette-Kuntz, H., Lloyd, J.E., Kasmara, L., Holden, J.J., & Lewis, M.E. (2008). Trends in autism prevalence: diagnostic substitution revisited. *Journal of Autism and Developmental Disorders, 38,* 1036–1046.

Copeland, W.E., Angold, A., Costello, E.J., & Egger, H. (2013). Prevalence, comorbidity, and correlates of DSM-5 proposed disruptive mood dysregulation disorder. *American Journal of Psychiatry, 170,* 173–179.

Cross, J.H., & Neville, B.G. (2009). The surgical treatment of Landau-Kleffner syndrome. *Epilepsia, 50,* Suppl 7, 63–67.

Curatolo, P., Paloscia, C., D'Agati, E., Moavero, R., & Pasini, A. (2009). The neurobiology of attention deficit/hyperactivity disorder. *European Journal of Paediatric Neurology, 13*, 299–304.

Dale, R.C., & Heyman, I. (2002). Post-streptococcal autoimmune psychiatric and movement disorders in children. *British Journal of Psychiatry, 181*, 188–190.

Debes, N.M., Hjalgrim, H., & Skov, L. (2009). The presence of comorbidity in Tourette syndrome increases the need for pharmacological treatment. *Journal of Child Neurology, 24*, 1504–1512.

Dopheide, J.A., & Pliszka, S.R. (2009). Attention-deficit-hyperactivity disorder: an update. *Pharmacotherapy, 29*, 656–679.

Faraone, S.V., Sergeant, J., Gillberg, C., & Biederman, J. (2003). The worldwide prevalence of ADHD: is it an American condition? *World Psychiatry, 2*, 104–113.

Fernell, E., & Ek, U. (2010). Borderline intellectual functioning in children and adolescents—insufficiently recognized difficulties. *Acta Paediatrica, 99*, 748–753.

Fernell, E., & Gillberg, C. (2010). Autism spectrum disorder diagnoses in Stockholm preschoolers. *Research in Developmental Disabilities, 31*, 680–685.

Fernell, E., Hedvall, A., Norrelgen, F., Eriksson, M., Höglund-Carlsson, L., Barnevik-Olsson, M., et al. (2010). Developmental profiles in preschool children with autism spectrum disorders referred for intervention. *Research in Developmental Disabilities, 31*, 790–799.

Fernell, E., Hedvall, Å., Westerlund, J., Höglund Carlsson, L., Eriksson, M., Barnevik Olsson, M. et al. (2011). Early intervention in 208 Swedish preschoolers with autism spectrum disorder. A prospective naturalistic study. *Research in Developmental Disabilities, 32*, 2092–2101.

Ghuman, J.K., Arnold, L.E., & Anthony, B.J. (2008). Psychopharmacological and other treatments in preschool children with attention-deficit/hyperactivity disorder: current evidence and practice. *Journal of Child and Adolescent Psychopharmacology, 18*, 413–447.

Gillberg, C. (1983). Perceptual, motor and attentional deficits in Swedish primary school children. Some child psychiatric aspects. *Journal of Child Psychology and Psychiatry, 24*, 377–403.

Gillberg, C. (1995). *Clinical child neuropsychiatry*. Cambridge: Cambridge University Press.

Gillberg, C. (2009). Developmental and neuropsychiatric disorders of childhood. In: J. Aicardi (Ed.), *Diseases of the nervous system in childhood* (3rd ed.). London: Mac Keith Press.

Gillberg, C. (2010). The ESSENCE in child psychiatry: early symptomatic syndromes eliciting neurodevelopmental clinical examinations. *Research in Developmental Disabilities, 31*, 1543–1551.

Gillberg, C., & Coleman, M. (2000). *The biology of the autistic syndromes* (3rd ed.). London: Cambridge University Press.

Gillberg, C., & Kadesjö, B. (2003). Why bother about clumsiness? The implications of having developmental coordination disorder (DCD). *Neural Plasticity, 10*, 59–68.

Gillberg, C., & Söderström, H. (2003). Learning disability. *Lancet, 362*, 811–821.

Gillberg, C., Ehlers, S., Schaumann, H., Jakobsson, G., Dahlgren, S.O., Lindblom, R, et al. (1990). Autism under age 3 years: a clinical study of 28 cases referred for autistic symptoms in infancy. *Journal of Child Psychology and Psychiatry, 31*, 921–934.

Gillberg, I.C., Gillberg, C., & Ahlsén, G. (1994). Autistic behaviour and attention deficits in tuberous sclerosis: a population-based study. *Developmental Medicine and Child Neurology, 36*, 50–56.

Hill, A.L., Degnan, K.A., Calkins, S.D., & Keane, S.P. (2006). Profiles of externalizing behavior problems for boys and girls across preschool: the roles of emotion regulation and inattention. *Developmental Psychology, 42*, 913–928.

Hagerman, R.J., Berry-Kravis, E., Kaufmann, W.E., Ono, M.Y., Tartaglia, N., Lachiewicz, A., et al. (2009). Advances in the treatment of fragile X syndrome. *Pediatrics, 123*, 378–390.

Howlin, P. (2008). Autism and diagnostic substitution. *Developmental Medicine and Child Neurology, 50*, 325.

Iacoboni, M. (2006). Failure to deactivate in autism: the co-constitution of self and other. *Trends in Cognitive Sciences, 10*, 431–433.

Kadesjö, B., & Gillberg, C. (1999). Developmental coordination disorder in Swedish 7-year-old children. *Journal of the American Academy of Child and Adolescent Psychiatry, 38*, 820–828.

Kadesjö, B., & Gillberg, C. (2000). Tourette's disorder: epidemiology and comorbidity in primary school children. *Journal of the American Academy of Child and Adolescent Psychiatry, 39*, 548–555.

Kadesjö, B., & Gillberg, C. (2001). The comorbidity of ADHD in the general population of Swedish school-age children. *Journal of Child Psychology and Psychiatry, 42*, 487–492.

Kadesjö, C., Hägglöf, B., Kadesjö, B., & Gillberg, C. (2003). Attention-deficit-hyperactivity disorder with and without oppositional defiant disorder in 3–7-year-old children. *Developmental Medicine and Child Neurology, 45*, 693–699.

Keen-Kim, D., & Freimer, N.B. (2006). Genetics and epidemiology of Tourette syndrome. *Journal of Child Neurology, 21*, 665–671.

Klin, A., Volkmar, F.R., Sparrow, S.S., Cicchetti, D.V., & Rourke, B.P. (1995). Validity and neuropsychological characterization of Asperger syndrome: convergence with nonverbal learning disabilities syndrome. *Journal of Child Psychology and Psychiatry, 36*, 1127–1140.

Kopp, S., Kelly, K.B., & Gillberg, C. (2010). Girls with social and/or attention deficit: a descriptive study of 100 clinic attenders. *Journal of Attention Disorders, 14*, 167–181.

Law, J., Tomblin, J.B., & Zhang, X. (2008). Characterizing the growth trajectories of language-impaired children between 7 and 11 years of age. *Journal of Speech, Language, and Hearing Research, 51*, 739–749.

Lundervold, A.J., Posserud, M.B., Ullebø, A.K., Sørensen, L., & Gillberg, C. (2011). Teacher reports of hypoactivity symptoms reflect slow cognitive processing speed in primary school children. *European Child & Adolescent Psychiatry, 20*, 121–126.

Mahone, E.M., & Hoffman, J. (2007). Behavior ratings of executive function among preschoolers with ADHD. *Clinical Neuropsychologist, 21*, 569-586.

Miniscalco, C., Westerlund, M., & Lohmander, A. (2005). Language skills at age 6 years in Swedish children screened for language delay at 2(1/2) years of age. *Acta Paediatrica, 94*, 1798-1806.

Miniscalco, C., Nygren, G., Hagberg, B., Kadesjö, B., & Gillberg, C. (2006). Neuropsychiatric and neurodevelopmental outcome of children at age 6 and 7 years who screened positive for language problems at 30 months. *Developmental Medicine and Child Neurology, 48*, 361-366.

Minnis, H., Rabe-Hesketh, S., & Wolkind, S. (2002). Development of a brief, clinically relevant, scale for measuring attachment disorders. *International Journal of Methods in Psychiatric Research, 11*, 90-98.

Minnis, H., Green, J., O'Connor, T.G., Liew, A., Glaser, D., & Taylor, E. (2009). An exploratory study of the association between reactive attachment disorder and the attachment narratives in early school-age children. *Journal of Child Psychology and Psychiatry, 50*, 931-942.

Monk, C.S., Peltier, S.J., Wiggins, J.L., Weng, S.J., Carrasco, M., Risi, S., et al. (2009). Abnormalities of intrinsic functional connectivity in autism spectrum disorders. *NeuroImage, 47*, 764-772.

Moretti, G., Pasquini, M., Mandarelli, G., Tarsitani, L., & Biondi, M. (2008). What every psychiatrist should know about PANDAS: a review. *Clinical Practice and Epidemiology in Mental Health, 4*, 13.

Mulligan, A., Anney, R.J., O'Regan, M., Chen, W., Butler, L., Fitzgerald, M., et al. (2009). Autism symptoms in attention-deficit/hyperactivity disorder: a familial trait which correlates with conduct, oppositional defiant, language and motor disorders. *Journal of Autism and Developmental Disorders, 39*, 197-209. Erratum in: *Journal of Autism and Developmental Disorders, 39*, 210-211.

Niklasson, L., Rasmussen, P., Oskarsdóttir, S., & Gillberg, C. (2009). Autism, ADHD, mental retardation and behavior problems in 100 individuals with 22q11 deletion syndrome. *Research in Developmental Disabilities, 30*, 763-773.

O'Brien, G. (2006). Behavioural phenotypes: causes and clinical implications. *Advances in Psychiatric Treatment, 12*, 338-348.

Ollendick, T.H., Jarrett, M.A., Grills-Taquechel, A.E., Hovey, L.D., & Wolff, J.C. (2008). Comorbidity as a predictor and moderator of treatment outcome in youth with anxiety, affective, attention deficit/hyperactivity disorder, and oppositional/conduct disorders. *Clinical Psychology Review, 28*, 1447-1471.

Pinkhardt, E.H., Kassubek, J., Brummer, D., Koelch, M., Ludolph, A.C., Fegert, J.M., et al. (2009). Intensified testing for attention-deficit hyperactivity disorder (ADHD) in girls should reduce depression and smoking in adult females and the prevalence of ADHD in the longterm. *Medical Hypotheses, 72*, 409-412.

Pliszka, S.R. (2000). Patterns of comorbidity with attention-deficit/hyperactivity disorder. *Child and Adolescent Psychiatric Clinics of North America, 9*, 525-540.

Rasmussen, P., & Gillberg, C. (2000). Natural outcome of ADHD with developmental coordination disorder at age 22 years: a controlled, longitudinal, community-based study. *Journal of the American Academy of Child and Adolescent Psychiatry, 39,* 1424–1431.

Rourke, B.P. (1988). Socioemotional disturbances of learning disabled children. *Journal of Consulting and Clinical Psychology, 56,* 801–810.

Sadiq, F.A., Slator, L., Skuse, D., Law, J., Gillberg, C., & Minnis, H. (2012). Social use of language in children with reactive attachment disorder and autism spectrum disorders. *European Child & Adolescent Psychiatry, 21,* 267–276.

Saemundsen, E., Ludvigsson, P., & Rafnsson, V. (2008). Risk of autism spectrum disorders after infantile spasms: a population-based study nested in a cohort with seizures in the first year of life. *Epilepsia, 49,* 1865–1870.

Sharp, S.I., McQuillin, A., & Gurling, H.M. (2009). Genetics of attention-deficit hyperactivity disorder (ADHD). *Neuropharmacology, 57,* 590–600.

Shaw, P., Lalonde, F., Lepage, C., Rabin, C., Eckstrand, K., Sharp, W., et al. (2009). Development of cortical asymmetry in typically developing children and its disruption in attention-deficit/hyperactivity disorder. *Archives of General Psychiatry, 66,* 888–896.

Sikora, D.M., Pettit-Kekel, K., Penfield, J., Merkens, L.S., & Steiner, R.D. (2006). The near universal presence of autism spectrum disorders in children with Smith-Lemli-Opitz syndrome. *American Journal of Medicine Genetics. Part A, 140,* 1511–1518.

Skuse, D.H. (2009). Is autism really a coherent syndrome in boys, or girls? *British Journal of Psychology, 100,* 33–37.

State, M.W., Pauls, D.L., & Leckman, J.F. (2001). Tourette syndrome and related disorders. *Child and Adolescent Psychiatric Clinics of North America, 10,* 317–331.

Stores, G. (2006). Sleep disorders. In: C. Gillberg, R. Harrington, & H-C. Steinhausen (Eds.), *A clinician's handbook of child and adolescent psychiatry.* Cambridge: Cambridge University Press.

Strang-Karlsson, S., Räikkönen, K., Pesonen, A.K., Kajantie, E., Paavonen, E.J., Lahti, J., et al. (2008). Very low birth weight and behavioral symptoms of attention deficit hyperactivity disorder in young adulthood: the Helsinki study of very-low-birth-weight adults. *American Journal of Psychiatry, 165,* 1345–1353.

Swanson, J.M., Wigal, T., & Lakes, K. (2009). DSM-V and the future diagnosis of attention-deficit/hyperactivity disorder. *Current Psychiatry Reports, 11,* 399–406.

Swedo, S.E., Leonard, H.L., Garvey, M., Mittleman, B., Allen, A.J., Perlmutter, S., et al. (1998). Pediatric autoimmune neuropsychiatric disorders associated with streptococcal infections: clinical description of the first 50 cases. *American Journal of Psychiatry, 155,* 264–271.

Vaughan, B., Fegert, J., & Kratochvil, C.J. (2009). Update on atomoxetine in the treatment of attention-deficit/hyperactivity disorder. *Expert Opinion on Pharmacotherapy, 10,* 669–676.

Wing, L. (2005). Reflections on opening Pandora's box. *Journal of Autism and Developmental Disorders, 35,* 197–203.

Volkow, N.D., Wang, G.J., Kollins, S.H., Wigal, T.L., Newcorn, J.H., Telang, F., et al. (2009). Evaluating dopamine reward pathway in ADHD: clinical implications. *Journal of the American Medical Association, 302,* 1084–1091. Erratum in: *Journal of the American Medical Association, 302,* 1420.

Wright, A.J., King, M.J., Wolfe, C.A., Powers, H.J., & Finglas, P.M. (2010). Comparison of (6 S)-5-methyltetrahydrofolic acid v. folic acid as the reference folate in longer-term human dietary intervention studies assessing the relative bioavailability of natural food folates: comparative changes in folate status following a 16-week placebo-controlled study in healthy adults. *British Journal of Nutrition, 103,* 724–729.

Zeanah, C.H., Keyes, A., & Settles, L. (2003). Attachment relationship experiences and childhood psychopathology. *Annals of the New York Academy of Sciences, 1008,* 22–30.

Prevalence of ADHD, DAMP, and ESSENCE

To be able to assess the meaning of the high population rate of ADHD, DAMP, and all the other ESSENCE, one must have an idea of how common behavioral abnormalities and learning difficulties are in the general population of children, adolescents, and adults.

It is estimated that, in many Western countries, between one in four and one in six of all children who start school have such a degree of behavioral problems that some form of supportive/treatment measure is believed to be called for. In the Nordic countries, many of these children will eventually come into contact with Child and Adolescent Mental Health Services (CAMHS)/child psychiatry or pediatric/neuropediatric units. The highest rate is found in large cities where, at least in Sweden, between one in four and one in six have been in contact with CAMHS at some point growing up. In other countries, where child psychiatry services may be less well developed or less accessible, rates of attendance will, of course, usually be lower.

Teachers estimate that around one in five to one in six of all children have such learning difficulties that extra supportive measures should be taken. Of these children, around one in 10 have an IDD with an IQ below 70, and many have BIF with an IQ below 85. Around onethird of all with any kind of learning difficulties have dyslexia.

ADHD

The rate of ADHD is generally agreed to be somewhere in the range of 4% to 8% of all schoolchildren (Faraone et al., 2003). Probably about half this proportion is recognizable already in the preschool years. These "preschool cases" are possibly among the most severe and tend to be most persistent, and most of these remain impaired by ADHD, ADHD symptoms, or other consequences of the disorder in adult age.

In adults, most studies suggest that the prevalence is a little more than half of that in school-age children—that is, around 3% to 4% (Biederman et al., 2011). These figures would suggest that slightly less than half of all individuals who meet diagnostic criteria for ADHD in childhood "grow out of" ADHD before (or early in) adult age. This is probably too simplistic a view, and most of the evidence indicates that (some, including sometimes quite severe) ADHD symptoms will remain for life even in individuals who no longer meet full diagnostic criteria for impairing ADHD.

Up until recently, the male-to-female ratio in ADHD was reported to be in the range of three to one or even higher. However, studies on adults suggest that females with ADHD have often been missed from the point of view of "correct" diagnosis in childhood and come to the attention of specialists only after adolescence. A recent Swedish study of school-age girls indicated that the vast majority of girls with ADHD are missed for many years in childhood or misdiagnosed as suffering from "only" depression, anxiety, and/or family relationship problems (Kopp et al., 2010). Women with "personality disorder," "chronic fatigue," or "chronic pain syndromes," according to a number of recent studies, often have an early childhood history and ongoing symptoms of ADHD.

The diagnostic criteria for ADD/ADHD have changed several times over the past three decades, which has caused problems when it comes to providing exact figures regarding the population rate. When the DSM-IV was published, the number of diagnosed and treated cases of ADHD increased dramatically, and it is currently under discussion whether we should expect an even higher prevalence rate of the disorder under the DSM-5 (Batstra & Frances, 2012).

The overlap between ADHD and DAMP is, by definition, significant. Around half of all children diagnosed with ADHD have comorbid DCD and would therefore meet the diagnostic criteria for DAMP, if they were only examined thoroughly enough in terms of motor control and perception that such a diagnosis would be possible to determine. This is rarely the case in most countries where ADHD is a widespread concept, and the diagnosis of DCD (and hence DAMP) is rarely made. It is worth mentioning yet again that ADHD symptoms are *always* present in cases of DAMP. It is possible that *some* motor/perceptual symptoms always occur in cases of ADHD, but this has not yet been researched in an entirely satisfactory manner. A conservative conclusion is that ADHD (severe and milder forms) affects about one in 15 children and that on one end of this spectrum motor/perceptual problems are very pronounced, in the middle both motor/perceptual problems and attention problems are pronounced, and on the other end attention problems are predominant.

In cases of ADHD there is significant comorbidity—that is, there is a very high rate of coincidental ("non-ADHD") problems of different kinds, including learning difficulties and a variety of mental health disorders. Conclusions in this area are, however, complicated by the fact that up until the arrival of the DSM-5, the DSM system has not supported ADHD diagnoses being given in cases where, for example, a diagnosis within the autism spectrum has already been given. The exclusionary nature of many of the DSM diagnostic categories has meant that the true rate of associated conditions and disorders in the whole field of neuropsychiatric/neurodevelopmental disorders has been grossly underrated. The very few studies that have actively neglected the exclusion criteria of the DSM have found comorbidity rates of about 85% in ADHD in general population samples and of 65% to 100% in different types of clinical samples (Kadesjö & Gillberg, 2001).

DCD

About 5% of all school-age children meet criteria for DCD (Kadesjö & Gillberg, 1999), and about half of this group have severe ADHD as well (with much of the link between the two being accounted for by shared genes) (Martin et al., 2006). DCD/motor perceptual dysfunction is, by definition, always present in cases of DAMP (see below). In addition, a few percent of all 6- to 7-year-olds have DCD without having ADHD (and thus without meeting the criteria for DAMP). DCD seems, just like DAMP and ADHD, to be about three times more common among boys than among girls. However, one study of 100 girls referred to clinics because of social and/or attention deficits indicated that DCD may be much more common in girls than previously understood.

DAMP

In a survey of all 6- to 7-year-olds in Gothenburg, Sweden, during the mid-1970s the rate of DAMP (ADHD with concomitant DCD) was estimated at 4.0% to 7.1%. In a similar study in Skaraborg, western Sweden, during the mid-1990s the rate was estimated at 6.9%. In both studies—just as in a study from Karlstad, mid-Sweden, in the 1990s—there was some uncertainty and an interval of around 4% to 7% was indicated in which the "true" DAMP rate should reasonably be located. The results confirmed that at least one child in every Swedish school class had DAMP (ADHD with DCD). Severe DAMP occurred in approximately 1.5%, while moderate DAMP was about three times as common.

In several different studies there have been around three times as many boys as there have been girls with DAMP. However, some observations indicate that there could be more girls with DAMP problems, but some of them do not get diagnosed. One reason for this is that girls—even when problems exist—are less hyperactive and less violent, and their difficulties are therefore trivialized.

DAMP seems to be somewhat more common in areas with social problems, but it is unclear whether this is because possible associated problems, for example acting-out behavior, lead to the problems being discovered more often, or because the fundamental problems actually are more common.

Surveys on the subject up until now do not suggest that DAMP is any more common in large or medium-sized cities than in the countryside, as is the case with many more unspecified mental problems.

Studies regarding the prevalence of DAMP in younger and older children either are unavailable or have had such major flaws that it is not possible to draw any conclusions from them. There is much to suggest that it is difficult to determine with certainty whether children below the age of 5 should be diagnosed with DAMP if their difficulties are not extremely pronounced. In the same manner, it seems as though there are considerable difficulties giving a diagnosis from the age of puberty onward. The symptoms change so much over time—not least of which the motor problems and possible hyperactivity become less prominent—that it can be difficult to determine the diagnosis based on the current set of symptoms alone.

Around one in five individuals with DAMP have an IQ bordering on IDD. One in five have an IQ close to borderline intelligence (around 85 IQ). Around one in 10 people with DAMP are of above-average or exceptional intelligence (IQ above 115).

Three out of four persons with DAMP develop major reading and writing difficulties, and many of these have dyslexia. Other learning difficulties are also very common.

Slightly more than two out of three children with DAMP have psychiatric disorders such as depression, oppositional defiant disorder, conduct disorder, and autistic traits/autism spectrum disorders. Among those with severe DAMP, the group with autism spectrum disorders is very considerable (a bit over half of everyone). The majority of these will come into contact with CAMHS at some point during development. This, in turn, means that at least every fourth child examined and subsequently diagnosed at a CAMHS clinic would be likely to have DAMP.

ESSENCE

If one looks at the full range of neurodevelopmental disorders subsumed under the ESSENCE category (see Chapter 3, specifically Table 3.2), the general population rate of all these taken together would be on the order of 10% of all children being affected around the time of starting school. Probably only about half of this group—in some countries smaller or much smaller proportions—would be diagnosed and registered as having one or more of the specific named ESSENCE diagnoses (e.g., ADHD, ASD, IDD, SLI, Tourette syndrome). Boys would still be reported to represent around 75% of these, but the "real" rate is probably more like 65%, given that girls are generally missed altogether, are misdiagnosed, or will get their correct diagnosis only several years later.

CONCLUDING REMARKS

Around one in 10 children starting school in Sweden have ADHD, DCD, ASD, IDD, or Tourette syndrome (or combinations of these) or another major problem/disorder subsumed under the ESSENCE category. Around half of those with ADHD and about half of those with DCD meet criteria for DAMP (i.e., they meet criteria for the other of those two diagnoses if they meet the criteria of one of them), and a quarter within this group have severe DAMP. Boys are affected three times more often than girls. There is a highly significant degree of comorbidity, not least in terms of learning difficulties/academic problems and mental/psychiatric disorders. Some of the comorbidity (such as dyslexia following SLI and depression following ADHD) can be seen—at least partly—as secondary complications of the "invisible" disorder, whereas other comorbidity (including the connection with ASD and Tourette syndrome) is more likely to be a manifestation of more basic primary biological connections. ADHD/DAMP/ESSENCE is one of the major public health issues of our time.

REFERENCES

Batstra, L., & Frances, A. (2012). DSM-5 further inflates attention deficit hyperactivity disorder. *Journal of Nervous and Mental Disease, 200,* 486–488.

Biederman, J., Petty, C.R., Clarke, A., Lomedico, A., & Faraone, S.V. (2011). Predictors of persistent ADHD: an 11-year follow-up study. *Journal of Psychiatric Research, 45,* 150–155.

Faraone, S.V., Sergeant, J., Gillberg, C., & Biederman, J. (2003). The worldwide prevalence of ADHD: is it an American condition? *World Psychiatry, 2,* 104–113.

Kadesjö, B., & Gillberg, C. (1999). Developmental coordination disorder in Swedish 7-year-old children. *Journal of the American Academy of Child and Adolescent Psychiatry, 38,* 820–828.

Kadesjö, B., & Gillberg, C. (2001). The comorbidity of ADHD in the general population of Swedish school-age children. *Journal of Child Psychology and Psychiatry, 42,* 487–492.

Kopp, S., Kelly, K.B., & Gillberg, C. (2010). Girls with social and/or attention deficits: a descriptive study of 100 clinic attenders. *Journal of Attention Disorders, 14,* 167–181.

Martin, N.C., Piek, J.P., & Hay, D. (2006). DCD and ADHD: a genetic study of their shared aetiology. *Human Movement Science, 25,* 110–124.

Development of Symptoms During Childhood and Adolescence

DHD, DAMP, and the other categories subsumed under the ESSENCE umbrella imply disruptions of "normal" development. Children with ADHD/DAMP/ESSENCE develop much like other children, although not according to a similar curve, and not in all domains of functioning. Some difficulties diminish over the years; others become apparent only relatively late in the individual's development. This means that one cannot expect a symptom overview to be the same in cases of ADHD/DAMP regardless of the individual's age. The fact is that the symptoms vary markedly from one age period to another.

In the following, an overview of the "typical" symptoms encountered in children with ADHD and DAMP will be given. The list is long, but that is because the disorder is complex and because so many associated ("non-core") problems are present in virtually every case that comes to clinical attention.

PROBLEMS WITH ATTENTION, ACTIVITY, AND IMPULSE CONTROL

When discussing activity control problems and attention disorder, one first has to say something about how one defines the terms "attention," "activity control," and "impulse inhibition."

ATTENTION

"Attention" is a difficult term that, to an extent, has different meanings to different people and in different situations. It encompasses a variety of different aspects, reflected, for example, in terms such as "focusing of attention," "sustaining attention," "shifting of attention," and "joint attention" (Mirsky & Duncan, 2001).

Attention means that the brain's "receiving" functions—consciously or partly consciously—are directed toward specific phenomena within or outside one's own organism. Upon hearing a sound, one listens up; if one feels a sense of discomfort in one's stomach, one registers it/thinks about it; when one senses an object in the sky, one looks toward it. How long one can sustain attention and how flexible one is in the ability to shift attention determines, to a large degree, which perception of reality and self-image one will have. In some situations it is necessary to maintain one's attention on an object or an event in order to be able to get a complete enough idea of that thing or series of events. In other situations a significant flexibility in the ability to shift attention is required, so that one can be aware of several parallel processes without becoming confused. In a select few situations it is instead a great advantage to be rigid when it comes to shifting attention. A task that requires extreme concentration is easier to perform if one does not allow oneself to be distracted by other important, but for the task at hand irrelevant, information. It is thus not a given that flexibility is always better than rigidness where attention is concerned and hence it is not clear where the line for "attention *disorder*" should be drawn, either. As with most human functions, behaviors, and abnormalities/disorders, it is a matter of variations between different extremes, of dimensions rather than categories.

Attention is affected by a variety of partly correlated factors such as ability to concentrate, distractibility, ability to automate, short-term memory, "working memory," stamina, degree of activity, processing speed, ability to multitask, and alertness. These abilities and traits are, in turn, affected by such things as mood, unease/calmness, hunger/thirst, and physical well-being/disease.

One of the difficulties in determining what one actually means by attention and what the fundamental problem is in cases of ADHD/DAMP is the tendency of many doctors, psychologists, and teachers to not think of any exact meaning when using words such as "attention," "distractibility," and "ability to concentrate." They are often used as more or less synonymous terms for abilities and traits that we intuitively understand the meaning of but that we cannot define precisely. In a Swedish study there turned out to be low correspondence between different doctors regarding assessment of 6-year-old children as regards their (1) ability to concentrate, (2) distractibility, (3) activity level, and (4) ability to stay still. What one doctor defined as concentration difficulties was not interpreted in the same way by another. However, when one compiled the assessments of all four there was near-perfect concurrence: almost everyone who was perceived as abnormal within one of the four areas was also assessed as abnormal within one of the other four areas, although not always within the same. In other words, it seems as though the terms used (attention, concentration, distractibility, and so on) together denote an area of functions—intimately dependent on one another—that can be identified by most people but for which one does not necessarily use the same terminology to describe them. It is this area of functions that henceforth will be called attention. Attention deficit then naturally refers to a disorder within this area of functions.

Some people have no difficulties taking note of relevant information, but then find it hard to hold on to it and are easily distracted by irrelevant stimuli. In this case one will generally get the impression that the person has mild to moderate *concentration difficulties*. If, in addition, the person has problems with directing his or her attention in an appropriate manner, one would instead get the impression that there are extreme concentration difficulties present.

It is doubtful whether there is actually any essential or even significant difference between attention disorder and concentration difficulties. However, "concentration difficulties" is generally the term that teachers, parents, and children, adolescents, and adults with ADHD/DAMP choose themselves when they try to describe their difficulties in directing and sustaining attention. It is rare for laymen to characterize such difficulties as "attention disorder."

It is also difficult to distinguish "attention" functions from what is known as "executive functions" (Pennington & Ozonoff, 1996). Some specialists would see attention as being part of executive functions; others would distinguish the two and regard them as clearly separable. There is a more detailed discussion about executive functioning later in this chapter.

ATTENTION DISORDER

Children with ADHD generally (and particularly those who meet criteria for DAMP; that is, those who have coexisting DCD) have a very noticeable attention disorder. The disorder manifests in many different ways and it is as of yet unclear whether all the problems that are currently being chalked up to the attention disorder actually have anything to do with attention functions. Some of the most common terms used to describe the difficulties in attention are "concentration difficulties," "low stamina," "high or low distractibility," "difficulties in adjusting one's activity," "inability to stay still," "alertness problems," and "automatization problems."

Difficulties regarding concept of time (Smith et al., 2002), and possibly also short-term/working memory and processing speed are also generally viewed as closely related problems (Lundervold et al., 2012).

These days it is common for attention disorder and problems with overview and planning, impulse control, and concept of time to be classified under the umbrella term "executive function disorders" and thus viewed as symptoms of disorders in the function of the frontal lobes (Diamond & Lee, 2011).

THE ATTENTION DISORDER "IN ITSELF"

In cases of attention disorder there are generally difficulties both in terms of directing one's attention to relevant information (e.g., to respond when someone calls one's name) and in terms of maintaining it for an appropriate amount of time. It is common for the person's attention to not be sustained long enough, but also for it not to be redirected quickly enough toward new information. In the former case the impression given will be that the person is not listening but instead jumping from one thing to another and seeming easily distracted, on edge, or nervous. In the latter case one will instead get the impression that the person commits fully to the task in an excessive manner, blocking out everything else and getting stuck in the activity at hand. This type of disorder also manifests as a reduced ability to listen or listen up/respond when spoken to.

When testing a person's attention in the context of a clinical examination, so-called go/no go tasks are often used wherein the subject is asked to, for example, push a button in conjunction with hearing a certain signal (e.g., two short chimes) and not to push it in conjunction with hearing another signal (e.g., one short chime). The signals are given in headphones and come at relatively short intervals. Attention ability is assessed by analyzing the reaction time (time between hearing the signal and pressing the button) and the number of missed button presses. Attention to visual stimuli can also be tested in the same fashion. The number of incorrect inputs gives an idea of the person's impulsiveness (Wehmeier et al., 2012).

ACTIVITY CONTROL

People are different when it comes to activity level, in terms of both mental activity and motor activity. It is well established that some children are motorically active and others considerably more passive, without them necessarily being considered abnormal. It is difficult to say exactly what the normal level is and hence also difficult to draw the lines for hyperactivity and hypoactivity. There is probably a "standard distribution" of the degree of motor activity among the population at all ages, which is to say that the majority are located relatively near the average level and only a few far from it, at either extreme. In rare cases, those who are located at either of these extremes are perceived as abnormal or "pathological" or as "cases" of hyperactivity or hypoactivity. At the extremes of this spectrum, one can also find people who have disorders and brain injuries, and who, for these reasons, are *pathologically* active or passive. The mildest of these latter cases are probably impossible to—based on symptoms—tell apart from those who are there "due to standard distribution."

A typically hyperactive child around, for example, the age of 3almost never stays still, moves about constantly, fidgets with anything and everything, and is often perceived as "nervous." It is as if the child were driven by a high-rpm motor. A typically hypoactive child of the same age almost constantly remains stationary and moves slowly, almost only if one prompts him or her to movement. At a higher age the hyperactivity can come to be perceived almost exclusively as nervousness and shows clearly through a constant fidgeting or drumming of the fingers and hands, rocking the legs or body back and forth, and a general restless behavior. Hypoactivity in adult years is almost generally synonymous with passivity, slowness, or even "laziness."

Everyone knows that almost all people can sometimes find themselves at either of these extremes but that they are most often located somewhere in between, in some kind of normal-active mode. We control and adjust our activity level in an automatic and intuitive manner so that it is adapted to the situation. This control sometimes occurs very consciously, but most of the time without us considering how it happens at all. During hard physical labor or in conjunction with practicing sports it is normal to be very motorically active. During a lesson, lecture, or deskwork it is normal to be motorically inactive. The ability to adapt to the current situation and maintain an appropriate degree of motor activity is crucial to whether we are perceived as normal-active or not. It is this activity *control* that is so often lacking in cases of ADHD/DAMP.

ACTIVITY CONTROL PROBLEMS

One of the most striking symptoms of ADHD/DAMP is the difficulty in modifying one's activity level so that it is appropriate in the current context.

Overactivity is fairly common, as demonstrated by both the U.K. (*hyperkinetic* disorder) and the U.S. (attention-deficit/*hyperactivity* disorder) diagnostic classification systems. Yet only about a third of all children with one of the diagnoses ADHD or DAMP clinically give the impression of being noticeably and constantly overactive in their wakeful state. When actometers (counters that register every motor movement in, for example, either leg)are used to measure the total motor activity over a whole day, it is in only a select few children with ADHD/DAMP that one has been able to determine a clearly elevated total motor activity.

However, alternating between hyperactivity and hypoactivity/passivity is a very common occurrence. This can give the impression of significant overactivity, even though the child's total activity during an average day is normal or even unusually low.

Hypoactivity occurs in perhaps every tenth child with ADHD/DAMP. In girls with ADHD/DAMP the rate of hypoactivity is probably higher. In this subgroup there is an especially large risk that the diagnosis may go undetected. It is difficult to detect underlying difficulties in attention and concentration in someone who stays still and does not cause problems in the classroom by running around all over the place or fighting.

IMPULSE CONTROL PROBLEMS

Almost half of all children with ADHD/DAMP are severely deficient in terms of impulse control. ADHD is, as has already been mentioned, split into three subgroups: one primarily lacking in concentration and attention, one that above all has a lack of impulse control and is overactive, and one that displays both attention deficit and hyperactivity/lack of impulse control.

Poor impulse control manifests in many different ways. Impulsiveness can be a typical ADHD symptom, even though it is important to remember that one can obviously be impulsive without having ADHD. Talking without addressing anyone in particular is also common. Extremely talkative children sometimes have the typical lack of impulse control that characterizes the impulsive variant of ADHD/DAMP. To act "on impulse," without thinking before hand, is common. It is perhaps even more common for there to be no interval between thought and action. Some children with ADHD/DAMP are described as demanding "immediate satisfaction of needs," something that is otherwise primarily characteristic of babies and children in their early preschool years.

In rare cases the poor impulse control is noticeable to no small extent as very severe aggressive outbursts and unpredictable explosive acts of violence. Such acts are sometimes encountered in children and adolescents with intermittent "attacks" of severely violent behaviors, which may be diagnosed under the label of "intermittent explosive disorder." There is a major risk that such actions are triggered in an impulsive boy with ADHD/DAMP who is constantly misunderstood, demeaned, teased, and ridiculed.

POOR EMOTIONAL REGULATION

What has just been stated about the rare occurrence of severe aggressive outbursts and how it may be associated with impulsivity is probably true also of the emotional dysregulation. This inability to regulate emotions and temper is now more and more often seen as not just a common symptom in ADHD, and perhaps associated with impulsivity, but maybe even as a core feature of the disorder. Inability to control temper is usually taken to be a symptom/sign of ODD, but some studies (Kadesjö, C., et al., 2003; Retz et al., 2012) indicate that it is an almost universal symptom in ADHD both in children and adults. In a Swedish study "inability to control temper" was actually *the* most common individual symptom of all in a large group of preschool children with a diagnosis of ADHD (with or without ODD).

Losing temper and constantly feeling "on edge," "nervous," "labile," "driven by a motor" are all typical of ADHD but are often misinterpreted as a separate emotional disorder such as generalized anxiety disorder.

LOW STAMINA

Reduced ability to sustain attention is described by many as low stamina. Sometimes low stamina is clearly associated with a generally low energy level, and the impression given is that of a tired or "lazy" person. It can also be portrayed as "seeming to be always bored" (although this impression can equally attach to those with ADHD who are impulsive and hyperactive). Other times an experienced low energy level can be present in someone with general overactivity or a shifting degree of activity and then often remains undetected.

DISTRACTIBILITY PROBLEMS

The majority of children with ADHD/DAMP are easy to distract. They are easily diverted from their current task and bothered by different kinds of irrelevant stimuli. This increased distractibility can in some cases also be described in terms of difficulties in sustaining attention, but other times one will see that their attention can be sustained relatively well as long as there are not any disruptive elements involved. The typical neuropsychological test setting is just such a situation, when there is structure and very little in the way of distracting features. Distractibility can therefore often be underreported if one goes only by what has been found during testing.

Other people with ADHD/DAMP have major problems with shifting their attention and are—once they have started working on a task—unable to let it go and move on to something else. This type of distractibility problem is especially characteristic of severe DAMP problems with autistic traits.

INABILITY TO STAY STILL — "ANTS IN THE PANTS"

Children with ADHD often feel a jittery sensation throughout their whole body, which they are completely unable to control and which makes them constantly move about in their chair, wiggle their toes, stamp their feet, move in place back and forth, pull and almost tug at their shoulders, chew on their tongue or some object, and grimace. They give the impression of having ants in the pants, or actually running about inside their whole body. Sometimes it is difficult to distinguish their almost constant motions from tics of different kinds. Conversely, many people who have tics and Tourette syndrome also have exactly the inability to stay still that is considered typical of ADHD.

ALERTNESS PROBLEMS, HYPERSOMNIAS, AND NARCOLEPSY

Reduced sleep and irregular sleep patterns are characteristic of many children with ADHD/DAMP (and other ESSENCE for that matter) during the first years of life. Sometimes such problems eventually turn into an almost increased need for sleep or at least a tendency to want to sleep more and more often than people of the same age.

Some children, perhaps particularly those with severe DAMP, have such a markedly fluctuating activity level over the course of a given day and at the same time such an obviously varying alertness that this in itself can constitute the greatest problem. Sometimes an overactive child with ADHD/DAMP can wind down fairly abruptly, become almost immobile, and then fall asleep. Most of the time the child manages to get to a couch or bed before falling asleep, but sometimes sleep hits him or her in such a sudden and overwhelming manner that it becomes difficult to distinguish it from narcolepsy (see Chapter 7). Hypersomnias of various kind are possibly overrepresented in the whole ESSENCE "population."

Some researchers argue that the fundamental problem in ADHD/DAMP is abnormally low alertness. There is scientific evidence supporting that low alertness in the nervous system can cause high—probably compensatorily high—motor activity. One could say that the body is trying to keep going so that the brain will not fall asleep. The low alertness as a cause of overactivity and activity without much aim or structure could be compared to a situation when one for some reason has slept too little for several days and then tries to go to sleep. One would often have major difficulties unwinding and would engage in an aimless activity that by others would almost be perceived as meaningless overactivity. Low alertness and overactivity/physical unrest along with associated problems also commonly occur among older people with reduced circulation in the brain. They often find it hard to settle down in the evenings, when the alertness and circulation in the brain are reduced. They sometimes become motorically overactive. A cup of strong coffee, which increases the person's alertness, can cause the body to settle down and ensure that the person has no trouble falling asleep.

Finally, one can compare this to treatment with stimulants, which often brings about a normalization of the activity level in overactive children; those substances raise the alertness in the nervous system while simultaneously reducing the person's motor activity.

AUTOMATIZING PROBLEMS

A common problem among the majority of the different functional disorders that are present in cases of DAMP (and possibly in ADHD without DCD also) is the difficulty in automating. It can be a matter of difficulties in automatically performing a set movement pattern, such as repeatedly jumping on one leg without having to think about how to go about it or repeatedly twisting one's hand back and forth in a fluent manner (Kadesjö & Gillberg, 1999). There can also be problems with standing on one leg while talking to someone or quickly accessing memorized facts, for example if someone asks for the name of a well-known person.

Most of us manage—after practicing for a while—to perform familiar action patterns and mental activities without thinking actively about what we are doing. We cross the street without thinking, "I'm crossing the street now." We eat with our mouths closed without thinking, "Keep your mouth closed, keep your mouth closed" for every bite. We converse in a casual manner without needing to have total mental control of the whole situation at all times. A lot of what we do is handled automatically without the need for constant reflection.

Children with DAMP (and many with ADHD without DCD) almost always have problems with automation. They find it hard to perform tasks that demand repetition in a persistent manner. For them to manage such tasks, they need to constantly think about exactly what they are doing. Anyone will realize that it must be tiresome to think "close your mouth" for every bite. Neither is it hard to understand that the ability to multi-task suffers if one cannot manage to let any of these things be handled automatically. If one constantly has to think about everything one does—how to stay still, how to walk straight ahead, how to eat with one's mouth closed—it is obvious that the ability to multitask suffers. It should also be apparent that one can easily get exhausted and that one may seem to have low stamina or simply be bored.

It is yet unclear what the word "automation" entails in a neurophysiological sense. Metaphorically one could liken it to a relatively quickly rotating lighthouse beacon located centrally in the nervous system, a beacon that quickly enough lights up the area or the functional circuits in the brain that need to be activated in order for the specific function/information that at that moment is to be performed/conveyed without the need for higher centers to get involved and make decisions. Perhaps many of these children's problems within different areas could simply be a result of deficits in their automation ability. This issue is addressed further in Chapter 10.

PLANNING DIFFICULTIES AND POOR "EXECUTIVE FUNCTION"/EXECUTIVE FUNCTION DEFICITS

Poor ability to get an overview and problems with distinguishing different sequences in a chain of events and the chronological relationship between them are very common in cases of ADHD, with or without DCD. Difficulties in predicting and planning often end up being a result of these problems but can also exist in cases where one cannot document the other difficulties. Poor impulse control surely also plays a part. Typical of children with this type of problems is to take on new tasks without thinking, without a plan. For precisely this reason they also get into difficulties with homework and various school assignments. Teaching children with ADHD/DAMP to plan is among the most important things in a well-thought-out intervention program.

The planning difficulties are generally part of what is nowadays usually referred to as "executive dysfunction." *Executive functions* are often defined as the mental characteristics that enable us to maintain a strategy over time (seconds, minutes, hours, weeks, or longer) in order to reach a goal that is not within immediate reach.

Executive functions can also be seen as an umbrella term for all cognitive processes that regulate, control, and manage other cognitive processes, including planning, working memory, problem solving, verbal reasoning, inhibition, mental flexibility, task switching, and initiation and monitoring of actions (and, according to some, attention "in itself").

The *executive system* is a theorized cognitive system that controls and manages these other cognitive processes. It is responsible for processes that are sometimes referred to as "executive functions," "executive skills," "supervisory attentional system," or "cognitive control." It is generally agreed that the prefrontal areas of the frontal lobe are necessary but not sufficient for carrying out these functions. It is becoming gradually accepted that the cerebellum is also intimately involved in some of the processes controlled by the executive system.

Children with ADHD/DAMP (and many of those with other ESSENCE as well) have major problems almost across the board with this type of executive function. Both "attention" and "working memory" (ability to hold on to the different thoughts required to perform a task) are important aspects of the ability to maintain a strategy. Some researchers distinguish between executive functions, attention, and working memory, whereas others include all of them in the same category.

POOR SENSE OF TIME

Many children with ADHD/DAMP and other ESSENCE have a poor sense of time (Smith et al., 2002). This does not necessarily mean that they cannot tell time or that they have difficulties with, for example, having an idea about the length of minutes, hours, and days, even though such difficulties are common. The typical scenario is that they do not have any natural sense of time and cannot intuitively determine whether a long or short period of time has passed. These problems regarding sense of time lead to major secondary concerns: children, adolescents, and adults with ADHD/DAMP often arrive late, they do not notice when time passes, they start working on their assignments too late or are tormented by the feeling of not knowing how much time remains. Some try to structure their time in an almost obsessive-compulsive manner by using clocks, schedules, and reminders of different kinds—and this can, indeed, sometimes be a very useful way of dealing with the problem.

The poor sense of time is sometimes a consequence of the difficulty in distinguishing sequences in chains of events and the deficits in planning ability that result from it ("executive dysfunction"). At other times the absence of sense of time leads to something that comes across as poor planning despite the fact that a plan may very well have existed—it is just not possible to realize since the person's idea of how much time has elapsed is not consistent with actual real-life conditions.

In severe cases of ADHD/DAMP it is not uncommon to not be able to "tell time" in one's late teens or young adult years. The difficulties in learning how to tell time are especially major when it comes to non-digital clocks. This is generally a result of a combination of problems: visual perception difficulties, abstraction difficulties, and poor sense of time. The problems can be hard to detect, perhaps above all because one has difficulty believing that it can exist among adults with normal intelligence.

Difficulties regarding concept of time, and also short-term/working memory and processing speed, are also often viewed as closely related problems. Individuals with ADHD have problems discriminating the duration of tasks. Neurocognitive findings of timing deficits in ADHD are furthermore supported by functional neuroimaging studies that show dysfunctions in the key inferior fronto-striato-cerebellar and fronto-parietal networks that support timing functions (Noreika et al., 2012).

GROSS MOTOR SKILL DIFFICULTIES

The term "gross motor skill difficulties" refers to problems with large physical movements. The difficulties can manifest as general motor clumsiness, balance problems, and difficulties learning how to ride a bicycle, swim, ski, skate, and handle a ball.

The vast majority of everyone with DAMP (and many of those with ADHD without concomitant DCD) perceived themselves as motorically clumsy during their childhood. In general this clumsiness has also been apparent to the people around them, but sometimes it has been hidden by, for example, an attention disorder and an associated lack of adequate fear, or "foolhardiness" if you will. The clumsiness is made up of one or more of the following components: poor automatism, low muscle tone (hypotonia), balance problems, motor coordination difficulties, and abnormal motor control.

Automation Problems

Much like in every other area of ADHD/DAMP, automation deficits are one of the most important underlying mechanisms behind clumsiness in terms of gross motor skills. Motions can sometimes be performed smoothly, even perfectly, but upon repeating them, automation deficits make the movements look clumsy. This easily leads to the idea that "he can probably manage if he just puts his mind to it," which is true to some extent; he could in fact manage for a short while if he were to direct all his energy and attention toward it.

Low Muscle Tone

At least half of all children with ADHD/DAMP have low or very low muscle tone (hypotonia), provided they do not direct all of their attention toward increasing it, in which case it can reach normal levels for a short while (Rasmussen et al., 1983). This mild to moderate muscular hypotonia results in "hyper flexibility" in joints, poor physical posture—primarily general weakness, protruding stomach, large lower back, and dragging gait—but also open mouth, a tendency to drool, breathing that sounds like snoring, and difficulties keeping a firm grip when writing by hand or eating with a knife and fork.

Balance Problems

Just shy of half of all children with DAMP (and many with ADHD without DCD) have overt balance difficulties. This can, among other things, contribute to "high anxiety," fear of heights (including standing on ladders, walking up staircases), and difficulties learning how to ride a bicycle. Some people with ADHD (particularly those who also have DCD and meet criteria for DAMP) do not want to sit on stools or chairs without armrests, since they can experience balance problems or even "vertigo" if they do not feel support from either side.

Motor Coordination Difficulties

It is difficult for many children and adults with ADHD/DAMP to coordinate body movements smoothly. This is not due to just poor automation skills, but also difficulties doing different things with the right and left or upper and lower halves of the body. It can be hard to manage alternating jumps and more particular jumps like jumping with one's right arm held forward and right leg backward, left arm backward and left leg forward. By the same token there are often major difficulties in differentiating and assigning movements so that they are made in only, for instance, the wrist or fingers; frequently, several other joints are needlessly involved (e.g., elbow and shoulders and sometimes even the joints of the jaw). Some children and adults have major accompanying oral motions every time they try to write something with a pencil.

For many children—and certain adults—with DAMP (and probably this is more to do with the DCD than the ADHD part of the condition), the inability to plan motor actions seems to be a crucial problem.

Movements and actions are performed without having been planned in a logical sequence first. This can result in several different movements being performed more or less at the same time when they were in fact supposed to be carried out in a certain order, one after the other. This gives a chaotic and clumsy impression, even though none of the individual parts of the movements can be described as clumsy or abnormal.

Abnormal Motor Control

In approximately 20% of all cases of DAMP (and maybe about 10% of all in the population who meet the criteria for ADHD), motor control is clearly abnormal or "damaged." These are cases where the person's motor control (e.g., in the legs) deviates in the same manner as in cerebral palsy, but to a lesser extent. In such cases it can sometimes be difficult to determine whether the diagnosis is most consistent with cerebral palsy or DAMP/DCD. The tendon reflexes (e.g., the heel and knee reflexes) are sometimes clearly abnormal in these cases. This is otherwise uncommon in cases of DAMP. Neurological examination with a reflex hammer—without specifically investigating motor control—rarely provides any relevant information for the actual diagnosing of DAMP.

FINE MOTOR SKILL DIFFICULTIES

Fine motor skill difficulties primarily include precision problems in the fingers, hands, and face. Certain speech difficulties could in principle also be included in this group, but for the sake of providing a clearer overview, they are addressed in the same section as other speech and language problems.

Difficulties with Hand Motor Skills and Precision

Hand motor skill difficulties and poor precision in hand motor control is almost universal in cases of DAMP and in many patients of ADHD who

do not meet the full criteria for DAMP/DCD. This can manifest as difficulties holding a pencil or crayon in a natural manner, forming letters
and adhering to specifications or restrictions (e.g., on lined or checkered
paper), tying knots, and buttoning shirts. Some children with such difficulties painstakingly work up time-consuming precision for such tasks,
but the majority are instead viewed as sloppy. Major difficulties at the din-
ner table and bad table manners are common, including poor judgment
of the force and angle required when, for instance, one is pouring water
from a pitcher (Pereira et al., 2001). Children, adolescents, and adults with
DAMP/ADHD almost always spill food and make a mess when they eat.
The fact that their clothes are often full of stains makes this especially easy
to notice.

Oral Motor Skill Difficulties

One problem not given its due attention is that children with DAMP/
ADHD have difficulties with oral motor skills and precise mouth and
facial movements. Many have trouble eating with their mouth closed,
others drool, and a number have difficulties articulating. Difficulties performing separate movements in the right and left half of one's face are
also common—for instance, blinking only on the right side or pulling the
left corner of one's lip over to the left. One's whole facial motor control
can seem fairly blank, perhaps due to poor innervation of the muscular
system in the face. This can in turn easily be misconstrued as a symptom
of depression with inhibited psychomotor activity. This assessment can
possibly be made more difficult by the fact that depression is a common
complication in cases of ADHD/DAMP.

PERCEPTION DIFFICULTIES

Perception difficulties include problems with visual, auditory, tactile, and
kinesthetic perception.

Auditory Perception Problems

Difficulties in auditory perception (perception of sounds/hearing) are likely the most common form of perception disorder in children with ADHD/DAMP (Gillberg et al., 1982; Rasmussen et al., 1983). It can be a matter of difficulties pinpointing where sounds originate—whether the sound came from the left or the right, from behind or in front of them—and determining the volume of a given sound or singling out distinctive, new, or "important" sounds among a general "buzz" of sounds. Many children with ADHD/DAMP have extreme difficulties picking up what is said by someone when there is a general "buzz" around them. When this problem is applied to a classroom situation it is easy to see why children find it hard to catch what the teacher is saying whenever the room is not absolutely silent (and how often is that the case?). Another auditory perception problem that is very characteristic of people with ADHD/DAMP is difficulty in "auditory feedback"—that is, when one does not automatically hear whether one is speaking loudly or softly and therefore cannot adjust one's tone of voice to fit the situation or conversation.

Phonological awareness problems, often associated with dyslexia, are perhaps actually best grouped with auditory perception disorders; however, they are instead addressed along with speech and language disorders below.

It is easy to imagine these auditory perception disorders causing major problems in everyday life. If one perceives a strong sound as weak or a sound as coming from the left when it is actually coming from the right, it is impossible to react in an appropriate manner in, for example, a dangerous situation. If one cannot discern that someone is calling one's name simply because others nearby are speaking in a normal tone of voice, one will naturally not react appropriately.

Visual Perception Problems

Difficulties in visually (with eyesight) distinguishing forms and distances and the locations of objects in the room are characteristic of many people with ADHD/DAMP (Rasmussen et al., 1983). It makes it difficult to, for instance, limn (draw) complex figures, letters, and numbers or to determine if a car is dangerously close or how far one has to stretch one's arm to reach a glass in the kitchen cabinet.

The difficulties in visual perception are often difficult to clearly define and distinguish from those in fine motor skills, or even the problems with gross motor skills. The term "visuomotor" problems is therefore often used when there are difficulties in, for instance, copying figures and imitation, as well as hand motor skills.

People with DAMP often have sprawling, childlike, excessively large or small, undriven, and "ugly"/illegible handwriting. The reasons for this may be problems with visual perception, hand motor skills, or automation—or combinations of these.

Tactile Perception Problems

For some children, adolescents, and adults with ADHD/DAMP, difficulties in using touch to determine the form and texture of various objects constitute a major problem. Such tactile perception disorders can cause problems when, for instance, one has to reach into one's pocket for a coin and there are other objects there as well. These difficulties most likely also contribute to fine motor skill difficulties due to the fact that there is no quick, adequate feedback of sensation to make motorical centers in the brain respond appropriately.

Kinesthetic Perception Problems

Difficulties determining the location and "direction" of one's own limbs are examples of kinesthetic perception difficulties that cause problems in terms of, say, the assessment of one's proximity to objects or other people. As a result of this, one can easily bump into people or become too heavy-handed, or walk right into walls or even mirrors. Without any ill intentions one may literally step on someone's foot, which could naturally wind up triggering conflicts, with verbal abuse or fighting as a result.

"Sensory Integration" and Synesthesias

Much as in other areas of ADHD/DAMP, there is a frequent occurrence of combinations of problems in terms of perception. It is rare for someone with ADHD/DAMP to exhibit isolated visual perception difficulties. However, one often encounters individuals with ADHD/DAMP who have both visual and auditory disorders and sometimes people with disorders within all four mentioned categories as well.

The integration of information from the various sensory channels is often impaired, and this, of course, leads to difficulties reacting in appropriate ways to sensory stimuli. For instance, an accelerating (noisy) car might be moving in the child's visual field from left to right, and this information may be processed correctly visually, but the child's auditory perceptual problem would lead the child to look in the opposite direction, in spite of the visual information telling him to follow the moving car with his gaze from left to right.

Some children in the ESSENCE group have synesthesias—that is, combined sensory experiences resulting from activation of one sensory or cognitive pathway leading to automatic, involuntary experiences in a second sensory or cognitive pathway. This can be unproblematic, "neutral," and even pleasant but can sometimes cause major problems.

SPEECH AND LANGUAGE PROBLEMS

Speech and language problems in cases of DAMP include both delayed development and clear symptoms of subsequently lingering abnormalities in language, speech, and voice.

Delayed Speech and Language Development

At least half of all children with ADHD/DAMP and other ESSENCE have delayed speech development and generally also delayed language development (Gillberg et al., 1983). Many parents are concerned about the child's hearing and may seek help for this reason. They are generally told that their child's hearing is normal. The parent typically reports that the child does not listen/respond when called on. Some children seem to exhibit difficulties understanding spoken language up to around 2.5 years of age but then develop enough spoken language to ease the parents' worries.

In one study, when testing the subjects at 4 years of age, as many as 60% still had sufficiently delayed speech development for it to be mentioned in the child clinic's medical record. However, upon follow-up six months later the language development was generally so much better that further check-ups were not deemed necessary.

Even though language development thus kicks off in most cases before the age of 5, many people experience delayed development far into their school years, although at that age it becomes much harder for a layman to detect this delay. After all, the child speaks and comprehends relatively well what is said to him or her. However, subtleties are easily lost, both in terms of the child's comprehension of them and his or her own ability to express them. Their vocabulary is limited and their grammar often very immature.

Grammar Problems

A large majority of all children with severe DAMP have significant problems with grammar (Rasmussen et al., 1983). Perhaps half of those with mild to moderate DAMP have similar albeit less pronounced problems. Some of these difficulties create problems with using referring expressions and forming sentences. Other times the abnormalities are similar to those seen in autism, with tendencies for echolalia, jumbling of pronouns, and repetitive questions.

Poor Vocabulary

Limited vocabulary, which is characteristic of just over half of everyone with ADHD/DAMP, is actually most apparent during the first years of life, but rather frequently causes the most difficulties starting in lower or upper secondary school. It is at this later age that one expects children to be able to express themselves in a nuanced manner. Children with ADHD/DAMP instead often use only a small number of words that they feel adequately familiar with and can use without running the risk of making a mistake. Their sentences are often filled with various empty words such as "like," "you know," "kinda," "sorta," or embellishing words or curse words. This is, of course, common among children in general, but it is on average considerably more pronounced in cases of ADHD/DAMP. Sometimes excessive use of curse words and other "foul language" can be a signaling symptom of Tourette syndrome (see Chapter 8).

The person's limited vocabulary can remain a problem in adulthood. Lots of words that the majority can take for granted as part of their vocabulary can lack meaning to someone with ADHD/DAMP. Vocabulary problems must be detected early in life. Systematic training is necessary in order for chronic difficulties to be avoided (Lundberg 2002). Some people with ADHD/DAMP are so aware of their difficulties in this area that they develop either low self-esteem as a result or a paradoxical interest in words and languages.

Articulation Difficulties

A majority of all children with severe DAMP exhibit articulation difficulties and pronounce speech sounds in an immature or incorrect manner (for their age). These difficulties are often a symptom of underlying phonological awareness problems. The problems are generally most apparent during the preschool years. Later in life these problems can be replaced by a conscious or unconscious tendency to express themselves in a slightly unclear or even slurred manner.

Phonological Awareness Problems

More than half of all children with DAMP in their school years have significant phonological awareness problems. This means that they find it hard to discern the differences between different speech sounds. Phonemes are the smallest speech sounds we make when we speak. The word "dad" contains three phonemes (d, a, d); the letter "L" contains two (e, l). Breaking down words into their smallest parts is hard or even impossible for anyone who has difficulties with phonemes—or phonological awareness problems.

Most evidence suggests that the phonological awareness problems are present long before the start of school and that they contribute to the difficulties in developing spoken language. In school they are probably the most important reason why reading and writing difficulties are so common in cases of DAMP. Phonological awareness problems naturally also increase the risk of pronunciation and articulation problems. Someone who finds it hard to tell the different sounds apart obviously also has difficulties pronouncing them. The person's speech can, as previously mentioned, become slurred. The "slurriness" can then become more pronounced when the person grows older and realizes that the underlying difficulties can be concealed to some extent by slurring past them, so to speak.

Abnormal Prosody

At least onethird—but probably a great deal more—of those with ADHD/DAMP exhibit abnormal prosody. Their voice is often monotonous and their prosody tends to go up and down in unusual or even incorrect places. This can in turn result in people around them having trouble understanding what they actually mean. Children and adults who have the combination of ADHD and autism/Asperger syndrome are almost always affected by this type of problem.

Abnormal Voice Quality

Children with ADHD often sound more or less chronically hoarse. People with DAMP often have a croaky, almost raspy tone of voice. It is also common for their voice to fluctuate both in volume and quality, which in turn can make it difficult for the person to whom they are talking to listen. Some people with DAMP constantly speak much too loudly—occasionally much too softly—for the situation at hand. Some of these abnormalities in voice qualities should most likely be possible to trace back to the auditory feedback problems previously mentioned in the paragraph on auditory perception disorders.

Pragmatic Problems

Some children with severe DAMP, although rarely those with mild to moderate DAMP, find it hard to use their language skills in a natural manner when socializing with other people. These pragmatic problems (i.e., difficulties using the knowledge one has in a natural, everyday, "practical" context) are very similar to those seen in an even more pronounced form in autism. They do not intuitively know when it is time to say something or how to start and maintain a conversation with someone. They do not understand that there is a risk of others growing bored if one launches into a long monologue or that others may not have the same information or knowledge as themselves. They can also have great difficulties understanding metaphorical expressions. They can misunderstand abstract expressions and questions and interpret them in a very concrete manner and may not understand, for instance, that the statement "Can you help me?" is not just a question that should be answered with a "yes" or "no" but also an indirect request for help. The children with severe DAMP who also exhibit autistic traits generally have major pragmatic problems.

Other Speech and Language Problems

Stuttering and "speeding speech" occur at an increased rate in cases of DAMP. The stuttering can sometimes be of an obsessive-compulsive nature and can be a partial phenomenon in Tourette syndrome. "Speeding speech" means that the words are spoken so quickly that it is hard for the person listening to discern what is actually being said.

THE FIRST YEAR OF LIFE

On the basis of clinical experience and parent retrospective reports, it is probably reasonable to divide ADHD/DAMP into three subgroups based on behavior during the first year of life. One of these is overactive and "messy" almost from the start. The second type is quiet or well behaved or "normal" until approximately age 1 to 18 months. In the third, there is no indication that anything is amiss or unusual at all.

The information available about the first year of life is primarily derived from retrospective studies (Gurevitz et al., 2012). Children generally get their ADHD/DAMP or other ESSENCE diagnosis—at the earliest—around 2.5 to 7 years of age, and reports of what they have been like and how they have behaved several years earlier are then often based on subjective memories, which do not necessarily provide a completely accurate description. Information of a prospective (looking ahead) nature is rarely available. All of this means that the information available about DAMP during the first year of life must be deemed as preliminary.

The Overactive Group

Almost half of all children with ADHD/DAMP exhibit abnormalities in terms of sleep, feeding, and activity level right from the first 12 months of life. This group is sometimes described as "early-onset hyperactive." Low sleep requirement, irregular sleeping habits, difficulties sucking, excessive voracity, "bellyache," proneness to screaming, and constant motor activity are characteristics typical of many children within the group. Their breathing is sometimes irregular and their airways are soft, with tendencies for snoring and panting.

Their level of motor activity can be so high that it can even become difficult for one person alone to change the child's diapers; the child's arms and legs may move around so much that there may be a need for two people to hold the baby so that the diaper can be put on.

It is fairly common for children within this group to start walking at a very young age, as early as 8 to 10 months old. Their actual walking "skill" may not be excellent, and many fall over and tumble; perhaps bruises and other injuries occur. One suspects that the child is not quite ready to handle an activity as advanced as walking, but that the high activity level, being prone to impulses, and "foolhardiness" are behind the need to quickly move around on two legs instead of on all fours. There is a widespread view that being able to walk at an early age indicates general early development, but unfortunately this is not true. It can be seen as an indication of a positive development outlook only if it coincides with early development of social and language skills. Starting to walk very early (before 10 months of age) should probably rather be regarded as a potential symptom of ADHD.

Early-onset extreme overactivity is often a partial phenomenon in different/overlapping disorders, including ASD, bipolar disorder, Tourette syndrome, epilepsies, and severe intellectual disability. It is always necessary to consider the possibility of these conditions before settling on the possibility that it probably is a matter of ADHD.

The Quieter Group

Many children with ADHD/DAMP have been "perfectly normal," "nice," or noticeably quiet during their first year of life. Unlike the overactive group there has fairly frequently been a suspicion of delay or disorder in the normal development. Some mothers express their concern at child clinics for this very reason.

It is not unusual for children within the quiet group to have had abnormalities in their motor behavior. Occurrences of rolling and banging one's head and rhythmically rocking back and forth on all fours have been observed in some cases. "Uhhhing" (i.e., rhythmically recurring "uhhh sounds") are relatively common, not least when the child is tired and especially when he or she is about to fall asleep. It is possible that these behaviors in some cases can constitute the first symptoms of Tourette syndrome or signal underlying autism problems.

Approximately every tenth child with DAMP is reported to have had motor stereotypies (recurring, stereotypical repeated physical movements) of different kinds, above all hand waving, toe-walking, and "excitement stereotypies," for example with the fingers stretched out over the mouth and nose.

Many children in the quiet group start walking significantly later than at 12 months of age.

Abnormal Modes of Movement

Aside from starting to walk at an extremely early age or, more rarely, at an unusually late age (after around 16 months), there are early symptoms of differing motor development in many children who later turn out to have DAMP.

Some children with ADHD/DAMP never crawl. Some of them move around by "dragging" their bottom across the floor or slithering around on their back or stomach; others get up directly from a seated position and start to walk without having been able to move on their own previously. Others roll around on their side or waddle around standing on all fours without performing any actual crawling movements.

ADHD/DAMP and other ESSENCE are relatively common among children who exhibit any of these kinds of unusual or abnormal modes of movement before they learn how to walk. Checking for abnormal modes of movement, including dragging one's bottom across the floor, is sometimes even used—along with other tests—as a screening criterion in cases where the question of DAMP is raised.

There is an unsubstantiated view that someone who learns how to walk without previously having crawled would then need to learn how to crawl afterwards. Normal development is assumed to require a crawling stage, and one cannot become "normal" if one has not experienced it. A number of more or less obscure forms of therapy when it comes to DAMP and similar problems are, among other things, based on this idea. There is no scientific evidence in support of these types of therapy; there is nothing to suggest that all people have to develop in the exact same way in order for them to become "normal."

Attentional Problems/"Not Listening"

A very observant parent, relative, or expert may note abnormalities in the attention of the child with ADHD right from the first year of life. Common occurrences include tendencies to not respond when others try to get one's attention and reduced ability to orient oneself toward "new events" in one's surroundings, as well as an excessive proneness to be disturbed by irrelevant stimuli. This can, of course, be hard to describe in these particular terms. Usually the person connected to the child reports that "something is different" or "something is wrong," without being able to pinpoint exactly what it is that is not working properly.

Autistic Traits

A group of children with severe ADHD (and just over half of everyone with severe DAMP) display symptoms during their first year of life that may lead one to consider the possibility of autism or autism spectrum disorder. It could be a matter of inability to listen/respond and show an interest in one's surroundings, but also of repetitive movements such as rocking one's body back and forth and stereotypical head-banging and waving one's hands around. Some children—although far from all of them—who exhibit these kinds of behaviors turn out to have lingering autistic symptoms.

Some parents wonder why their children seem so "unhappy" or even grouchy. These children are often part of the group that has a number of autistic traits in other areas as well. The American psychiatrist Paul Wender pointed out as early as 40 years ago that children with "MBD" suffered from "anhedonia," which is to say that they had a reduced ability to feel positive/negative emotional responses (or emotional rewards/ punishments, if you will) and excitement (including joy and sadness) in situations that would trigger these feelings in other children. It is possible that this "anhedonia" is an important, even central, problem in cases of ADHD/DAMP. Unfortunately there is as of yet limited research on this subject, not least due to the fact that it is difficult to find an appropriate research model for gathering information on anhedonia in toddlers.

THE PRESCHOOL YEARS

Inability to listen, delayed speech development, overactivity or a rapidly shifting degree of activity, and unfocused, "dreamy" attention are the most common obvious symptoms of ADHD/DAMP during the first years of preschool (Gillberg, 2010).

It is generally still possible to distinguish the overactive group from the quiet one around the beginning of the preschool years, but in many respects the two groups start to resemble one another so much during this period that the overall impression of them is dominated by similarities rather than differences, at least when the children are around 4 to 5 years old.

Concentration difficulties and shifts in activity level are typical of both subgroups from around the age of 2. Even the previously quiet group can during this time have periods of their day be dominated by overactivity or at least a varying activity level alternating between disorganized overactivity and passivity.

Children in the group with early overactivity generally give the impression of deviating more from the norm during their preschool years than those who were quiet in their first years of life. They usually come off as ill mannered and cause problems by being "foolhardy," "unruly," "mischievous," and almost impossible to have around in furnished rooms. They seem strangely unaffected by admonitions, reproofs, and encouragement. The aforementioned anhedonia makes its presence increasingly known.

The same tendency to not be affected in the same way as other children by reproofs and instructions exists within the quiet group as well. It is as if the child forgets whatever he or she is told. One moment the child is standing in front of his parent with an earnest look on his face, receiving an instruction, and upon being asked, "Did you hear what I said?" responds with a clear "yes"; the next moment it is as though the child had never heard what was said.

In both groups it is common for the parents to ask about the child's hearing at the child clinic or to contact an otologist (ear doctor), a phoniatrist (a type of speech doctor), or a speech therapist on account of delayed language or speech development. The rate of middle ear inflammation (otitis), inflammation of the Eustachian tube with or without fluid in the middle ear (otosalpingitis), and mild hearing impairments seems to be somewhat higher among children with DAMP than among children in the general population. This means that a relatively large amount of people with DAMP undergo ear operations, among others some that include the installation of drainage, or "tubes," in the ears. Sometimes this has a positive effect on language development, but there is generally no causal link between the mild hearing impairment and the delayed language development and thus the expected improvement may not occur. Also, most of the time, the parents are given reassuring words regarding the child's hearing. Eventually the child's language development starts to improve and the parents grow less concerned. Nevertheless, as previously mentioned, there still remain a number of language problems that are partly hidden behind the fact that the child does speak after all.

Toward the end of the preschool years the difficulties in fine motor skills and perception often become more noticeable. The child is unable to draw even a very simplified picture of a person, for instance one consisting only of a head (representing both the head and body) and legs/feet, at the expected age (around 3.5 to 4 years) and finds it hard to learn colors and concepts such as opposites and numbers. Even at age 5 the drawings come off as immature——that is, if the child even agrees to draw at all. Many children with DAMP refuse to draw, paint, and write or take part in any tasks at all that they find difficult. Unfortunately, this is generally viewed as defiance, laziness, or idiosyncrasy. One of the most common reasons why children do not want to participate in tasks or games that should be fairly appropriate for their age is that they know it would be too difficult for them. Refusing to participate is often a refusal to once again allow oneself to be publicly humiliated. The child can occasionally be seen practicing these tasks when they think nobody is watching.

The gross motor skills are usually also recognizable as clumsy, awkward, or otherwise abnormal toward the end of the preschool years. Until then, high activity level and lacking judgment have often been able to hide the difficulties that have actually been present. The child may have climbed up trees or up on roofs, and this has, understandably enough, been taken as an indication that his or her motor skills are normal. Upon closer inspection of children like that, however, one can see that their gross motor control is in fact clumsy, despite their daring nature. Some children with balance difficulties and clumsy motor control can actually have learned how to ride a bicycle and swim as early as the end of their preschool years. In these cases the child has often acquired the skill "by chance," for example when the bicycle has accidentally rolled down a slope with the child seated on it or when the child has fallen in the water and miraculously managed to stay afloat through various movements, which upon closer inspection do not resemble normal swimming motions all that much. The most common signs of problems with gross motor skills at this age are otherwise usually difficulties learning how to ride a bicycle and participate in various kinds of ball games, ice-skating, or skiing (on flat surfaces; they may fare better in slopes, since they produce a certain degree of momentum automatically). The difficulties are often most pronounced in the start-up phase: how is one supposed to make the bicycle gain speed and simultaneously maintain one's balance, how is one supposed to get one's ice skates on, maintain one's balance, and then also build up speed? The difficulties in attempting to master many things at once often become especially obvious when trying to teach the child with DAMP new motorical activities.

EARLY SCHOOL YEARS

For many children with mild to moderate ADHD/DAMP, who may have coped relatively well during their preschool years, starting school is the negative turning point. In school one is expected to be able to sit in a chair for many minutes at a time, concentrate on tasks that are not necessarily fun or interesting, and show interest in, as well as have what is needed for, learning how to read and write.

One must also be able to keep one's impulses in check, be quiet on command, listen up in certain situations, block out irrelevant stimuli, wait one's turn, and function in a group. Soon enough a certain measure of learning ability within a variety of different areas is expected as well—not just reading and writing—and many of these activities demand well-developed fine and gross motor skills and perception.

The problems fairly often become almost insurmountable as early as the first month of school, at least if the teacher is not prepared for the child's difficulties. A boy with ADHD, who in himself is often more active and aggressive than a girl with the same type of difficulties, is especially likely to cause problems in the classroom, right from the start. He cannot stay still, leaves his desk, disturbs his classmates, walks around the classroom, does not answer when spoken to, interrupts the teacher, and answers or says things without being asked. He looks out the window, rocks his chair back and forth, falls backward from his desk onto the floor, slams his desk lid right in the middle of an activity that requires silence, and may also be upset or almost inconsolably sad upon receiving even the slightest reprimand. He sometimes gets into fights after having, possibly completely inadvertently, shoved someone on his way into the classroom. The problems sometimes get even worse during recess. He scores an own goal while playing football, ignores the other children's problems, or "crashes" their games without noticing that he is annoying them. Soon he is known as someone one absolutely does not want near you during recess or in the classroom. He shows little interest in reading and writing, perhaps saying, "It doesn't interest me!," "I can't!," or "I don't want to!"

There is sometimes initially a great interest in reading and writing, which, however, quickly subsides when the learning difficulties grow more apparent and he is not given adequate help. His alertness fluctuates a great deal; sometimes the teacher finds him attentive and intelligent, but other times he conveys a half-asleep, "stupid," and lazy impression.

Before long, the problems risk resulting in a conflict between the teacher and the parents. The parents feel that the teacher shows little—or no—understanding. The teacher feels that the parents have failed in their effort to raise their child. Perhaps the teacher assumes that the domestic situation is filled with problems. If neither the parents nor the teacher know what is causing the child's difficulties, if neither of them have a name for the problems, there is a major risk that the child will be caught up in the middle of a battle of prestige between the parents and the school. It is easy to see how such a situation could exacerbate the child's difficulties adjusting.

When one or two years of school have gone by, it becomes obvious that the boy has reading and writing difficulties, possibly labeled as dyslexia. The motor control problems may have been recognized earlier on in PE class, but it is not uncommon for these to become highlighted as late as around the fifth year of school, even though they in actuality were most pronounced around the age of 7 or 8. Depending on which measures are taken, the learning problems may eventually eclipse the other problems more and more. It is also not uncommon for mental health problems, above all depression and conduct disorders with various kinds of adjustment difficulties, to dominate the symptom pattern, sometimes to the point where they are considered to be the primary issues. The DAMP problems can remain undiagnosed for many years, maybe forever.

Almost half of all children with ADHD/DAMP will come into contact with CAMHS during this period. The reason for this is often that one has misinterpreted the difficulties as being primarily of a psychological nature. There is no doubt that many of the symptoms that the child exhibits are secondary psychiatric effects of a primarily neurobiological disorder; the prominent problems are thus often of a psychological nature. Nor is there any doubt that, given these circumstances, that CAMHS should be the primary help institution. The problem is that there still exists a lack of information/education on the subject (e.g., within CAMHS), causing the child's difficulties to go undiagnosed. This may in turn result in parents and children feeling—rightfully so—misunderstood. Unfortunately there is thus a risk that the family's problems will be exacerbated and made permanent if the child's difficulties are not given their due attention.

Many children with ADHD/DAMP get no help whatsoever, neither with their dyslexia, their other learning problems, nor their motor control difficulties. Many also do not get any psychological help in dealing with declining confidence, depression, thoughts of suicide, adjustment problems, or conduct disorders. The relatively few who are provided with help with these difficulties are relatively often ultimately misunderstood, and the well-meaning effort to help ends up being misguided.

One should expect that half of all children with ADHD/DAMP are depressed around the age of 10 (Gillberg, I. C., 1985). Around the same number exhibit acting-out behaviors—that is, they fight, destroy property, and violate all manner of social norms for their age group (Kadesjö, C., et al., 2003). Quite a few of them smoke, get drunk, or participate in destructive gang activity. The overlap between depression and conduct disorder is significant. Around the age of 13 perhaps onethird have some kind of problems related to acting out. Depression is not as common as it previously was. Many who were previously depressed feel a little better at this point. Instead they come off as daydreaming and absent-minded, as though they were living "with their head in the clouds."

The motor control problems become less and less clinically significant over time in approximately two thirds of all people with ADHD/DAMP. This does not mean that their motor difficulties have just disappeared completely. Upon close inspection and demanding a higher measure of stamina and precision, the difficulties still come across as considerable. The general impression, though, is no longer that the child is clumsy in all of his or her activities.

The reading and writing difficulties, however, are only slightly lessened, at least if the child is compared with his or her peers. Employing good pedagogic methods leads to a very significant improvement in almost all cases, but relative to other children in the same age group, their problems are still very pronounced. Many children, and perhaps particularly many girls, who have the combination of ADHD and autism have reading and writing difficulties, but they may go unnoticed because clinicians believe that such problems rarely occur in individuals with autistic symptoms (Kopp et al., 2010).

In most cases the ability to concentrate improves—at least superficially—over the years. It is especially common for the overactivity—at least if it has been prominent—to subside. A significant deficit in attention could remain, though, quite often in combination with a significantly increased distractibility. An increased need for sleep is common during prepubescence. This generally stands in stark contrast to the low need for sleep and irregular sleeping pattern exhibited during the first years of life.

Girls with ADHD/DAMP sometimes have problems almost identical to those of boys with the same diagnosis, but other times their difficulties are much less obvious. Hypoactivity and social inwardness/withdrawal may hide a set of problems that are just as hindering, if not more so, as what one would find in boys. Boys with ADHD/DAMP almost always have problems that are apparent to anyone, among other things as a result of aggressiveness and elevated activity level; however, this is not to say that boys always get an actual diagnosis. Girls with ADHD/DAMP often have difficulties that are not equally obvious. They are neither correctly diagnosed nor are their difficulties given any attention in any other way. It is hard to decide which is worse: having one's problems recognized but incorrectly diagnosed or having them not be recognized at all. In the future, though, it is imperative that girls' difficulties within the DAMP spectrum be taken more seriously than they are today.

Both boys and girls with ADHD/DAMP tend to have their difficulties be most pronounced during their first years of school. It is over the course of these years that one risks laying the foundation of life-long low self-esteem—even in cases where the person would superficially seem to be exceedingly confident. It is also during these years that the most important preemptive efforts can be made. The fundamental disorder is generally hidden. This means that there is a maximum risk of impairment.

By discovering the basic problems and giving an appropriate diagnosis and adequate information, the degree of impairment can be significantly reduced. It is entirely possible to live with DAMP, provided that there is an understanding of the mechanisms behind the symptoms. This understanding must at the latest emerge during the early school years.

PUBERTY

Puberty can bring about major changes in children with ADHD/DAMP, positive as well as negative ones.

There is a belief, firmly rooted both among the general public and within school and health care institutions, that immaturity is an important cause of problems in childhood, not least among boys, and that someone who is immature will—as the word itself implies—eventually mature. Overactivity and learning problems are from this perspective viewed as signs of immaturity, and one expects them to subside and probably reach normal levels as the years go by.

A longstanding view with child and adolescent psychiatry, child habilitation, and school health care was that ADHD/DAMP and "MBD" improved during puberty and that the outlook—if secondary complications such as depression, acting out, and substance abuse could be prevented—would be exceptionally positive in almost every aspect. Unfortunately, in reality, things are not quite that simple. Admittedly, there does seem to be a smaller group of children with ADHD/DAMP who actually mature so much during their teens that one could almost describe it as having "healed," but a much larger group have lingering difficulties of some kind.

Part of the reason behind this inaccurate image of a very good outlook in cases of DAMP is that older studies have not emphasized connections between DAMP and dyslexia enough. It is already clear that motor control difficulties and problems with concentration and attention become less noticeable, if not more or less "healed," during the teen years. These observations initially led to an overly optimistic prognosis in cases of DAMP. Only when more and more studies showed a link between ADHD/ DAMP and dyslexia and other difficulties keeping up in school—and that such difficulties often persisted through puberty—did one draw the conclusion that the prognosis must often be regarded as uncertain.

Thus, some children with ADHD/DAMP mature in a very noticeable and positive manner during puberty. For a small group of these one could justifiably argue that puberty in itself has constituted an exceptionally positive period where virtually all severe symptoms of ADHD/DAMP have disappeared. Whether hormonal, neurophysiological, psychological, or other factors are behind this positive development is as of yet unclear.

For many people with ADHD/DAMP, puberty does not, in a relative sense, create any greater difficulties than it does for children without DAMP. Still, the fundamental difficulties in cases of ADHD/DAMP could—among other things due to the larger body, fuller voice, and (normally) increased proneness to aggressiveness, at least in boys—become more prominent during puberty than ever before. There is a major risk of conflicts arising between the child and parents, teachers, and friends.

For a small group of patients puberty seems to cause an actual exacerbation of the condition. A previously apparent case of borderline intelligence comes across more and more as pronounced IDD; the moderately clumsy motor skills seem almost disastrous and the overt perception disorders result in/lead to various kinds of psychotic symptoms. Perhaps around one in 15 people with DAMP develop a psychosis during their teens.

Also, the change from overactivity to underactivity in a considerable subgroup, combined with impulsive eating patterns, appear to lead to a very large increase in the risk of developing obesity in ADHD/DAMP. The rate of ADHD and ADHD-symptoms in pathological obesity is in the order of 40% (Hölcke et al., 2008).

CONCLUDING REMARKS

Children with severe ADHD/DAMP exhibit problems with (1) activity, impulse, and attention control and usually also (2) gross motor skills,

(3) fine motor movements, (4) perception, and (5) speech and language. Children with mild and moderate ADHD/DAMP exhibit problems with activity, impulsivity, and attention control and difficulties within one, two, or three, but not all four, of the other "ADHD/DAMP areas." The difficulties within every area of functioning can be of different kinds; this means that the symptoms can vary greatly from one child to another. In other words, ADHD/DAMP causes a heterogeneous symptom pattern.

The symptoms of abnormality within the different functional areas shift from one age to another, sometimes so much that it can be difficult to believe that it is still a matter of the same problems if one, for instance, met the child at age 6 and then did not see him or her again until around the age of 10. Not least is there a tendency for associated problems—such as dyslexia and various kinds of psychiatric complications—to become more and more dominant over the years. In such cases there is a considerable risk that the fundamental disorders are never properly diagnosed.

Some children with ADHD/DAMP see their condition improve before and during puberty, to the point where it can become difficult to recognize their original problems when they reach young adulthood. Many still have mild to moderate lingering symptoms, which manifest especially as oppositional and conduct problems (including alcohol and drug abuse), depression, academic failure, reading and writing difficulties, and other learning problems. A small group see their condition deteriorate during puberty, and some of these develop various kinds of psychoses.

REFERENCES

Diamond, A., & Lee, K. (2011). Interventions shown to aid executive function development in children 4 to 12 years old. *Science*, *333*, 959–964.

Gillberg, C. (2010). The ESSENCE in child psychiatry: Early symptomatic syndromes eliciting neurodevelopmental clinical examinations. *Research in Developmental Disabilities*, *31*, 1543–1551.

Gillberg, C., Rasmussen, P., Carlström, G., Svenson, B., & Waldenström, E. (1982). Perceptual, motor and attentional deficits in six-year-old children. Epidemiological aspects. *Journal of Child Psychology and Psychiatry*, *23*, 131–144.

Gillberg, C., Rosenhall, U., & Johansson, E. (1983). Auditory brainstem responses in childhood psychosis. *Journal of Autism and Developmental Disorders*, *13*, 181–195.

Gillberg, I.C. (1985). Children with minor neurodevelopmental disorders. III: Neurological and neurodevelopmental problems at age 10. *Developmental Medicine and Child Neurology, 27*, 3–16.

Gurevitz, M., Geva, R., Varon, M., & Leitner, Y. (2012). Early markers in infants and toddlers for development of ADHD. *Journal of Attention Disorders* (Epub ahead of print, June 28).

Hölcke, M., Marcus, C., Gillberg, C., & Fernell, E. (2008) Paediatric obesity: a neurodevelopmental perspective. *Acta Paediatrica, 97*, 819–821.

Kadesjö, B., & Gillberg, C. (1999). Developmental coordination disorder in Swedish 7-year-old children. *Journal of the American Academy of Child and Adolescent Psychiatry, 38*, 820–888.

Kadesjö, C., Hagglöf, B., Kadesjö, B., & Gillberg, C. (2003). Attention-deficit-hyperactivity disorder with and without oppositional defiant disorder in 3- to 7-year-old children. *Developmental Medicine and Child Neurology, 45*, 693–699.

Kopp, S., Kelly, K.B., & Gillberg, C. (2010). Girls with social and/or attention deficits: a descriptive study of 100 clinic attenders. *Journal of Attention Disorders, 14*, 167–181.

Lundberg, I. (2002). The child's route into reading and what can go wrong. *Dyslexia, 8*, 1–13.

Lundervold, A.J., Stickert, M., Hysing, M., Sørensen, L., Gillberg, C., & Posserud, M.B. (2012). Attention deficits in children with combined qutism and ADHD: A CPT study. *Journal of Attention Disorders* (Epub ahead of print, Aug. 31).

Mirsky, A.F., & Duncan, C.C. (2001). A nosology of disorders of attention. *Annals of the New York Academy of Sciences, 931*, 17–32.

Noreika, V., Falter, C.M., & Rubia, K. (2012). Timing deficits in attention-deficit/hyperactivity disorder (ADHD): Evidence from neurocognitive and neuroimaging studies. *Neuropsychologia* (Epub ahead of print, Sept. 28).

Pennington, B.F., & Ozonoff, S. (1996). Executive functions and developmental psychopathology. *Journal of Child Psychology and Psychiatry, 37*, 51–87.

Pereira, H.S., Landgren, M., Gillberg, C., & Forssberg, H. (2001). Parametric control of fingertip forces during precision grip lifts in children with DCD (developmental coordination disorder) and DAMP (deficits in attention motor control and perception). *Neuropsychologia, 39*, 478–488.

Rasmussen, P., Gillberg, C., Waldenström, E., & Svenson, B. (1983). Perceptual, motor and attentional deficits in seven-year-old children: neurological and neurodevelopmental aspects. *Developmental Medicine and Child Neurology, 25*, 315–333.

Retz, W., Stieglitz, R.D., Corbisiero, S., Retz-Junginger, P., & Rösler, M. (2012). Emotional dysregulation in adult ADHD: what is the empirical evidence? *Expert Review of Neurotherapeutics, 12*, 1241–1251.

Smith, A., Taylor, E., Rogers, J.W., Newman, S., & Rubia, K. (2002). Evidence for a pure time perception deficit in children with ADHD. *Journal of Child Psychology and Psychiatry, 43*, 529–542.

Wehmeier, P.M., Schacht, A., Ulberstad, F., Lehmann, M., Schneider-Fresenius, C., Lehmkuhl, G., et al. (2012). Does atomoxetine improve executive function, inhibitory control, and hyperactivity? Results from a placebo-controlled trial using quantitative measurement technology. *Journal of Clinical Psychopharmacology, 32*, 653–660.

Difficulties in Speech, Language, Reading, Writing, Mathematics, Motor Control, and Other "Specific" Learning/Developmental Disorders

Difficulties of any kind in reading and writing are reported by teachers in every fifth or sixth child between 7 and 13 years of age. About one in four of these have difficulties that are not proportional to factors such as general borderline intelligence or shortcomings in their education or home environment. These are the children who have what some call *dyslexia*. Specific difficulties in writing (dysgraphia) are found both in people who also have reading difficulties and as an isolated problem for a small group.

Major difficulties in mathematics are reported by teachers in at least one in 10 children between 7 and 13 years of age. About one in five of these have specific difficulties in mathematics, paralleling the problems with written language in those who have dyslexia. In these cases, the term *dyscalculia* is used.

Many children, both boys and girls, with ADHD/DAMP (and other ESSENCE) have difficulties in reading and writing (Åsberg et al., 2010;

Kadesjö, 2000). A large proportion of these have dyslexia. Dyslexia occurs 10 times more often in people with DAMP (in just under half of all) than it does in the population at large. Dysgraphia is almost a given if one has DAMP with dyslexia. Dyscalculia occurs in every fifth child with DAMP (and maybe about one in eight of those with ADHD)—that is, a rate very much higher than in the general population.

Virtually all children with both ADHD/DAMP and dyslexia have some form of problems with speech and language during their early childhood years (Rasmussen et al., 1983). A small group have problems with speech and language during their early childhood years but do not develop difficulties in reading and writing later on.

In DAMP, difficulties in motor control are inevitable because of the definition of the DAMP concept (DAMP = ADHD + DCD). In spite of this, when it comes to "specific" learning disability, the emphasis is not generally on the problems in motor control. Naturally, difficulties in motor control generate problems in physical education lessons; at least half of all children with DAMP have considerable difficulties in this area, but many of these go unnoticed and are therefore unable to get help.

The learning problems associated with DAMP in the areas of reading, writing, mathematics, language, and speech as well as motor control are some of the most important consequences or "comorbidities" of the fundamental disorder. There is, not least in these areas, a palpable risk of suffering from daily humiliation in school. It is this humiliation during classes in English, mathematics, and PE, to name only a few, that lays the foundation for the hatred of authority and society that, later in life, will characterize a small group of those with ADHD/DAMP. This is another example of why diagnosing and addressing "comorbid" difficulties must be done in an adequate manner.

SLI (SPEECH AND LANGUAGE IMPAIRMENT)

The speech and language problems that are often associated with ADHD/ DAMP, and that are always present in some form in cases of severe DAMP, were described in the previous chapter. They may not amount to a full diagnosis of SLI, but are, nevertheless, usually important for understanding the bigger picture in the individual case.

However, the following facts bear repeating: at least one in two children with DAMP have clearly delayed speech and language development; many have poor articulation; and grammatical problems and limited vocabulary are very common, even in teenagers and adults. A similar, but slightly less obvious, language and speech situation applies in ADHD without DCD.

Just over one in two children with severe DAMP have speech problems similar to those seen most prominently in people with autism. Some have echolalia, which means they repeat whatever is said to them, immediately or after a while. Others have a variant of this in which if they are asked a question, they whisper the question to themselves and then answer it. Palilalia also occurs in some people who also have tics and Tourette syndrome. Palilalia means that one repeats one's own sounds, words, or sentences one or more times consecutively.

The majority of children with ADHD/DAMP use their language in a social and flexible manner. A smaller group, once again mainly recruited from the group with severe ADHD/DAMP, have pragmatic problems that cause difficulties in initiating and maintaining a conversation, but also difficulties in understanding anything other than concrete meanings of spoken language. This group of problems is sometimes referred to as *semantic pragmatic disorder*, but *pragmatic disorder* is probably a more reasonable term, seeing as there are patients with severe pragmatic problems but without major semantic difficulties.

Phonological problems are, if not the rule, then in any case prevalent in people with ADHD/DAMP. In younger children these may appear as problems in articulation and pronunciation of different kinds. Later they may, outside of a specific test situation, be seen when the child finds it difficult or is even unable to rhyme and pick up on the rhythm of sentences or songs. It is possible that it is these phonological problems that underlie the high rate of dyslexia seen in children with ADHD (Gooch et al., 2011).

DYSLEXIA

Dyslexia occurs in almost half of patients with DAMP. The rate is probably considerably lower in those who have ADHD without DCD. Many more have difficulties in reading and writing that cannot be characterized as dyslexia (Miller et al., 2013). In total, eight in every 10 children with DAMP have some kind of problems in reading and/or writing (Gillberg, 2003). Children with severe DAMP virtually always have difficulties in reading and writing.

These difficulties are often detected even before the child starts school, manifesting as a lack of interest in words and letters and a diminished ability to learn—and comprehend—them if attempted. The problems generally become disabling during the first years of school, and it is common for children with severe ADHD/DAMP to not yet have learned to read by the end of year four (Gillberg, I.C., et al., 1983). Difficulties in forming letters using hand and pencil are also common.

Children with dyslexia who have low or lower than normal intelligence are generally spotted early on in school as, by and large, they do not learn to read or write at all. Some of these are incorrectly (most of the time) or correctly (in the odd case) perceived as having global intellectual disability/IDD. Problems can arise if they are placed in a special needs class, where they have difficulty identifying with other children who have overt mental retardation/IDD. Nevertheless, some of them still benefit from the special needs resources, whether through placement in a special school class or through resources reserved for extra support efforts in a "normal" class.

Highly intelligent people with ADHD/DAMP sometimes learn to read and write "on time," yet they still have difficulties. Their reading and writing do not develop at anything like the expected rate when factoring in intelligence, educational stimulation, and home environment. They may perform roughly on par with the class average all the way through lower secondary school, and this is perceived as "normal." The problem is that it is not normal when viewed in relation to their powers of reasoning, "speed of thought," and "general intelligence." Highly intelligent children with dyslexia almost always go around feeling stupid. They know that they think clearly and have original ideas, but when these are to be expressed in writing—sometimes even when they are to be expressed rapidly orally—things go awry. The problems become especially pronounced toward the end of secondary school, in college, and at university. It is clearly a major disadvantage to not be able to read and write quickly and without hindrance if one is to engage in theoretical studies. Add to this the deficits in attention and concentration and it becomes apparent how difficult it is for a young person with ADHD/DAMP to complete academic studies. This still does not deter some people from, for example, studying at university level. The price they pay, however, is having to constantly study diligently for exams and assignments during almost all of their free time.

ADHD/DAMP and dyslexia/difficulties in reading and writing are thus closely linked. Both mean chronic—often lifelong—disabilities. To live and grow with them one must acknowledge their existence and the fact that one most likely will not get rid of them, at least not completely. As with other disabilities one cannot run away from the problems by "taking time off" from them. Hence it is, unfortunately, generally destructive to take long breaks from reading and writing practice, during, for example, a long summer break. For someone who has DAMP and dyslexia and who does not spend any time at all on reading or writing during the summer months—albeit for the commendable purpose of finally taking a vacation from everything that is hard—there is a major risk that his or her performance will deteriorate when school starts up again during the fall term.

Dyslexia is also generally associated with language problems of different kinds (Miniscalco, 2006). Delayed speech development during one's preschool years is a very common precursor, and having a limited vocabulary in one's late teens a common resulting problem of this. In children, adolescents, and adults with dyslexia, it is always important to consider the possibility that ADHD/DAMP may simultaneously be present and also that language and speech functions may be affected. In other words, dyslexia is rarely an isolated condition. As much of a mistake as it has been in the past to not consider dyslexia and other learning disability in cases of ADHD/DAMP, just as much of a mistake could be made by not always being prepared to examine whether dyslexia may only be a symptom of a more complex problem encompassing activity control, attention, motor control, perception, and language/speech.

OTHER DIFFICULTIES IN READING AND WRITING

Major diagnostic problems sometimes arise in the case of children with difficulties in reading and writing who are of borderline intelligence or who have mental retardation/IDD. The most common reason for difficulties in reading and writing is likely to be just that, a lower than average IQ. If the child's level of intelligence is below the population average, one cannot expect his or her ability to read and write to be above or even at normal level. Half of all children are below the average intelligence for the population. One in six children have an IQ of less than 85 (i.e., below 85% of the average number for the age group in question). This is a plain fact that many people find hard to accept.

Society has found it difficult to accept that there are children with specific difficulties in reading and writing. In spite of this, there are now many who have now finally agreed to refer to such problems as dyslexia. It is considerably more difficult for society to accept that many children have "difficulties in reading and writing" simply because they are not of high or normal general intelligence. Over the past 50 years more and more "manual" jobs have disappeared. It has become more and more of a given that everyone has to study—and by "studying" one refers mostly to everything having to do with reading and writing. It is as though one would not be a complete person if one were unable to point to many years of literary studies. In a situation like this, it is obvious that many people with dyslexia, and even more with difficulties in reading and writing due to lower than normal intelligence, will be cast aside and fail in school and their working lives. This is one of the most important reasons why difficulties in reading and writing are claimed to be so common now, when they seemed to be rare half a century ago. A further complication that stems from the fact that the problems of many of those with difficulties in reading and writing are not recognized for what they really are, for example dyslexia or borderline intelligence, is that they gradually develop various mental problems, including depression and acting-out behaviors. At best the mental problems are finally detected, although they generally cannot be treated effectively if the fundamental problems, for example "ADHD," "DAMP," "DAMP with dyslexia," "dyslexia," or "borderline intelligence," remain unidentified.

DYSCALCULIA

Dyscalculia—or specific difficulties in mathematics—also occurs in a significant number of children with ADHD/DAMP. The rate of dyscalculia in the general population is estimated at below 3%, but some studies quote figures as high as one in 10 children (Ashkenazi et al., 2009; Butterworth et al., 2011; Shalev, 2004). It is at least as common in girls as in boys, and this contrasts with most neurodevelopmental disorders, which are much more common in boys. In people with DAMP and ADHD without DCD the rate is at least three, probably closer to 10, times greater ("NICE Guidelines," 2009). Some children have dyscalculia as well as dyslexia; others have an isolated, and in that sense "specific," impairment of their mathematical ability.

The mathematical difficulties can pertain to numbers and numeric concepts and, in such cases, may be much more complicated and difficult to remedy. Other times it is more a question of a circumscribed perceptual disorder, sometimes of a visual nature, for example when reversing numbers or turning them upside down. These disorders can often be ameliorated through systematic training, but in rare cases they can be very difficult to deal with or circumvent. Sometimes the difficulties in mathematics are, despite the description as "specific," only partial aspects of a more general problem with short-term and working memory. In such cases it is often the mental arithmetic that is made more difficult because of the difficulty in remembering several numbers at a time. Using pen and paper and a systematic method of calculation, which in itself can be difficult to learn to use, these kinds of difficulties in mathematics can usually be resolved relatively simply.

Quite a few children, adolescents, and adults with difficulties in reading and writing find mathematics to be relatively straightforward. If this is the case, then it is important to take note of and make use of it, since it can be one of the surest ways to a better self-esteem. However, it is important also to know that the difficulties in reading and writing can sometimes lead to "difficulties" in mathematics owing to the individual's inability to read the written math problems correctly or quickly enough, resulting in the person being unable to show his or her talent.

DIFFICULTIES IN MOTOR CONTROL

The difficulties in motor control inherent to DAMP were described in some detail in the previous chapter. Here it will only be mentioned that the fundamental problems are often made worse by the fact that there are "problems in learning of motor control," automatizing problems, and missed learning opportunities. The missed opportunities are, on the one hand, a result of children and adolescents with DAMP rarely being included when their peers are engaging in sports activities, and on the other, of how many—understandably enough—willingly avoid participating in physical education and sports or are simply relieved of such classes in school for medical/psychological reasons.

Overall there is, as in many other areas concerning ADHD/DAMP, a considerable risk of a vicious circle developing, wherein primary motor control difficulties lead to reduced practice and thus increasing motor problems in relation to one's peers. Unfortunately, there is no simple solution to this problem since it is often an accurate assessment by the child or the parents that one should avoid subjecting oneself to the bullying and teasing that clumsy children often have to endure. Good mental "health" and a sense of well-being and self-esteem are more important than possessing excellent motor skills. This becomes especially apparent upon reaching adulthood, when having excellent motor skills no longer carries the same high status that it does in childhood. On the other hand, there is of course the risk that the child's self-esteem will be affected negatively by the fact that he or she cannot cope with routine practical games or other activities. Decreased motor activity also means an increased risk of overweight and obesity (Hölcke et al., 2008). A good balance between the extremes of training and no training at all of motor skills is generally necessary.

CONCLUDING REMARKS

Reading and writing difficulties, including dyslexia, dyscalculia, and other "specific" learning problems, are the norm in ADHD/DAMP. For many individuals such difficulties overshadow everything from the time they start school. Teachers must receive adequate training on ADHD/DAMP and on the correlation between learning difficulties and attention problems so that the educational interventions can be adapted appropriately.

REFERENCES

Ashkenazi, S., Rubinsten, O., & Henik, A. (2009). Attention, automaticity, and developmental dyscalculia. *Neuropsychology, 23*, 535–540.

Åsberg, J., Kopp, S., Berg-Kelly, K., & Gillberg, C. (2010). Reading comprehension, word decoding and spelling in girls with autism spectrum disorders (ASD) or attention-deficit/hyperactivity disorder (AD/HD): performance and predictors. *International Journal of Language & Communication Disorders, 45*, 61–71.

Butterworth, B., Varma, S., & Laurillard, D. (2011). Dyscalculia: from brain to education. *Science, 332*, 1049–1053.

Gillberg, C. (2003). Deficits in attention, motor control, and perception: a brief review. *Archives of Disease in Childhood, 88*, 904–910.

Gillberg, I.C., Gillberg, C., & Rasmussen, P. (1983). Three-year follow-up at age 10 of children with minor neurodevelopmental disorders. II: School achievement problems. *Developmental Medicine and Child Neurology, 25*, 566–573.

Gooch, D., Snowling, M., & Hulme, C. (2011). Time perception, phonological skills and executive function in children with dyslexia and/or ADHD symptoms. *Journal of Child Psychology and Psychiatry, 52*, 195–203.

Hölcke, M., Marcus, C., Gillberg, C., & Fernell, E. (2008). Paediatric obesity: a neurodevelopmental perspective. *Acta Paediatrica, 97*, 819–821.

Kadesjö, B. (2000). [Pay attention to children with language development deviations]. *Läkartidningen, 97*, 3912–3913.

Miller, A.C., Keenan, J.M., Betjemann, R.S., Willcutt, E.G., Pennington, B.F., & Olson, R.K. (2013). Reading comprehension in children with ADHD: cognitive underpinnings of the centrality deficit. *Journal of Abnormal Child Psychology, 41,* 473–483.

Miniscalco, C. (2006). *Language problems at 2½ years of age and their relationship with school-age language impairment and neuropsychiatric disorders.* (Doctoral Thesis). Gothenburg University, Gothenburg.

NICE Guidelines (2009). Retrieved 15th January 2013, http://www.nice.org.uk/nicemedia/live/12061/42059/42059.pdf

Rasmussen, P., Gillberg, C., Waldenström, E., & Svenson, B. (1983). Perceptual, motor and attentional deficits in seven-year-old children: neurological and neurodevelopmental aspects. *Developmental Medicine and Child Neurology, 25,* 315–333.

Shalev, R.S. (2004). Developmental dyscalculia. *Journal of Child Neurology, 19,* 765–771.

Mental Health Problems/Additional "Psychiatric Disorders"

At least twothirds of all children with ADHD/DAMP (and other ESSENCE) develop impairing mental health problems while growing up. These impairments include those caused by disorders that are not encompassed by the definitions of ADHD or DAMP. In the United States, and to a certain extent in the United Kingdom, problems within the field of ADHD (attention deficit, hyperactivity, impulsiveness) are perceived as "mental disorders" and labeled in conjunction with psychiatric disorders, for example in the DSM-5. In the Scandinavian countries, ADHD/DAMP is often viewed more as a deviance from normal development and includes, apart from a number of behavioral symptoms, certain deviances in development of motor control, perception, learning, and speech/language. In accordance with this perspective, it is possible to have ADHD/DAMP with or without an additional psychiatric diagnosis. A few children with ADHD/DAMP are actually well adjusted both psychologically and socially and are relatively uninhibited by their disabilities in attention, motor control, and perception.

The most common additional psychiatric diagnoses in cases of ADHD/DAMP are depression, ODD, and conduct disorder (Thapar et al., 2012). Around 60% of all patients with ADHD/DAMP have had either one or both of these diagnoses before the age of 17 (Hellgren et al., 1994). Anxiety is also quite common but it is difficult to disentangle the symptom of anxiety both from ADHD as such (restlessness, "nervousness," irritability can be part both of ADHD and an anxiety disorder) and from depression.

Depression may be particularly common in mild or moderate cases of ADHD/DAMP. A minority of patients seem to have lasting problems with recurring depressions in their adult years. Some have conduct disorders that persist through adulthood, and many of these eventually develop an antisocial personality disorder and may end up involved in criminal activity.

In severe cases of ADHD/DAMP (and other ESSENCE), autistic traits are common instead. These are most apparent during the preschool years, when concern can arise as to whether the "correct" diagnosis really is autism. In some children with severe DAMP, the question often arises whether or not it might be a case of Asperger syndrome or atypical autism. There are also cases where children with severe "DAMP problems" during their preschool years ("ESSENCE") gradually show more and more of the typical symptoms of autism as time goes by.

A few children with ADHD are extremely hyperactive and impulsive even during their very first years of life. Children with autism, Tourette syndrome, bipolar disorder, and early-onset epilepsies, as well as some children with severe learning disability/intellectual developmental disorder can exhibit an equal, or even more pronounced, degree of hyperactivity during their first years. On occasion, tics occur in such children from about the age of 4 or later. Eventually the overall clinical picture of Tourette syndrome can become increasingly obvious, but generally not until the child has begun school.

It appears that different types of mental disorders with social phobia or social negativism become especially common from the late teens onward. In adult years there are quite a few, likely just under half, who, psychologically speaking, do fine and do not meet the criteria for a psychiatric diagnosis. In spite of this, their self-esteem is often poor or very poor. Some people with ADHD/DAMP, however, have, at least on the surface, an unusually well-developed self-esteem with little insight into the basic problems of their own disability.

DEPRESSION AND ANXIETY

Depression thus occurs very often in individuals with ADHD/DAMP. At least every other person diagnosed with DAMP has at some point during his or her formative years/development had so many symptoms of depression that the DSM diagnostic criteria for this disorder have been met.

In a small group of children and adolescents with ADHD/DAMP, the depressive symptoms are likely to be an indication of an early onset of depressive, or possibly manic depressive (bipolar), disorder with alternating periods of well-being and clear depressive episodes with depressed mood state.

In most people with ADHD/DAMP, it is, however, reasonable to interpret the depressive symptoms as a manifestation of the child feeling, after years of failures and constant complaints or open bullying, that life is hard, perhaps even not worth living, and that one's own body cannot handle things that others handle with ease. In the long run, without help and understanding, one cannot manage to convince oneself that one is "still good enough." With time, both energy and feelings of joy or well-being start to fade. Finally, all that is left is self-reproach, listlessness, and dejection.

Thoughts of suicide are not uncommon from around the age of 10 in children with ADHD/DAMP (Gillberg & Gillberg, 1989; Hinshaw et al., 2012). Among children without disabilities, thoughts of suicide are rare at prepubertal age. The exceptions to this are children who have been subjected to abuse or severe bullying of different kinds. Very few of children with ADHD/DAMP actually carry out suicidal acts, but it is still unsettling that almost 40% of all children with DAMP have contemplated suicide by the age of 10. There is no good evidence that ADHD medications are associated with an increased risk of suicide (McCarthy et al., 2009).

Depressive symptoms can appear at a very early age—sometimes they can be clearly distinguishable by the age of 3 or 4—and manifest as listlessness, "unhappiness" (a kind of general lack of joy as described earlier, which is otherwise uncommon in children), or "anhedonia." Some of these early-onset symptoms of depression are likely to be precursors of real depressive disorders.

It is far more common that the depressive symptoms surface only after the child has started school. The difficulties in reading and writing, suffered by many, soon contribute to a feeling of exclusion, of being different, of not being able to handle or cope with as much as the others and, hence, rapidly deteriorating self-esteem. As with children with other disabilities, for example children with cerebral palsy, it is common for the depressive symptoms to culminate around the age of 9 to 11. The reason for the high rate of depressive troubles at this particular age is most likely that it is not until that point that the child has the intellectual capacity and overview to be able to realize that his or her own condition constitutes a disabling problem and to identify it as abnormal. In the midst of all the depressive feelings, there is often also a strong element of anger. "Why has this happened to me, why does everything go so well for everyone else, why am I the only one who's failing?" are questions that many ask themselves, and they may direct their disappointment and anger toward themselves and their parents.

During puberty and the years leading up to it, a more resigned state of mind often emerges and it may become less apparent that the child/teenager is depressed. A slightly absentminded or daydreaming attitude is common instead. This may be the case more often among those with the mainly inattentive subtype of ADHD (="ADD").

A lowered general mood can remain after puberty. One in four people with ADHD/DAMP met the criteria for depression during their 17th year, according to the Gothenburg ADHD/DAMP study (Hellgren et al., 1994). Just under half of these had a depressive disorder. Apart from the ones with depression, many have low self-esteem. This can, however, not with certainty be seen as abnormal considering how many adults there are who do not have ADHD/DAMP and still have low self-esteem. Perhaps there is still a difference in the sense that adults with ADHD/DAMP (often associated with dyslexia, DCD, or borderline levels of intelligence) build their lacking self-esteem around the notion that they are "dumb" or stupid, which in turn is often connected to all the failures resulting from dyslexia (or the clumsiness or both). Depressive symptoms are common in adult life as well. Many women with a childhood history of ADHD—usually without a proper diagnosis of this disorder having ever been made—will be diagnosed by psychiatrists or general practitioners in adult life as suffering from depression, and it is very common in such circumstances for the "underlying" ADHD to be missed altogether.

Despite the rather bleak picture of the strong correlation between ADHD/DAMP and depression (Simon et al., 2013), it is important to emphasize that there is no inevitable connection, other than possibly within a small minority. With understanding and support it is likely that depression can be pre-empted, prevented, and alleviated. This is, however, assuming that the underlying difficulties are discovered and diagnosed.

It could also be the case that some degree of depression may also be a "healthy" sign in cases of ADHD/DAMP, at least during the early school years. If one recognizes one's difficulties—which is necessary for one to be able to take any concrete measures against them and to be able to learn to live with them—is it then not natural to, at least for a time, feel anger, disappointment, sadness, and dejection?

ANXIETY DISORDERS AND "DEMENTIA"

Many studies have indicated that anxiety is a common associated problem in ADHD (Bramham et al., 2012). It is unclear to what extent the full diagnostic criteria for an anxiety disorder are actually met, but, certainly, feelings of emotional unrest, a sense of "nervousness," being "high strung," and not being able to wind down and (in the evenings) go off to sleep are almost universal in ADHD at some stage of development (be it in the school years, adolescence, or adult age). Worries of various kinds are also common, and in some cases, clear attacks of panic or severe separation anxiety are present and functionally disabling.

In adult age, the nervous, high-strung, fidgety, unconcentrated presentation often leads adult psychiatrists, neurologists, and general practitioners to the—sometimes mistaken—notion that there must be an "underlying anxiety disorder." This would be particularly likely in patients not previously diagnosed with ADHD, and where the doctor consulted may not even reflect on the possibility of an underlying "primary" diagnosis of ADHD. Many adult women (and some men) who have not been diagnosed with ADHD in the early years may seek help for "nervous breakdown," "exhaustion," "feelings of being completely overwhelmed and not able to cope," inability to wind down in the evening, and sleep problems of various types. All this can be associated with various degrees of substance use disorder (alcohol, benzodiazepines, painkillers, or stimulants). Practitioners consulted will be likely to suggest diagnoses of generalized anxiety disorder (with or without depression), or panic disorder, or even "burnout syndrome," without first stopping to think whether or not ADHD could be part of the picture or, indeed in quite a number of cases, the only "real" disorder/problem.

In menopausal women, after the fertile period (when higher levels of estrogen and, hence, better regulated dopamine function in the brain have often controlled and—to an extent—concealed the symptoms of ADHD), there is often emergence of the same types of problems that were typical of the school-age years: executive function deficits, forgetfulness, lack of concentration, and sleep problems. In clinical practice, such women continue to be misunderstood by doctors who will diagnose (only) "menopausal syndrome," "generalized anxiety disorder," or "memory problems." Often in such cases, benzodiazepines are prescribed and referrals may be made for assessment of early signs of dementia. In women receiving estrogen therapy the symptoms may well subside, and many women recognize their much better executive functioning when receiving hormone therapies of this kind. The important bottom line in this context is that *all* women presenting from age 45 years and above with the types of problems outlined should be assessed with a view to discovering underlying ADHD. The best therapy they can hope to receive would be interventions known to be helpful for ADHD, not for anxiety disorder or depression or memory problems (or at least not *only* for such problems).

CONDUCT DISORDERS AND "ACTING OUT"

Conduct disorders, including ODD (see below) and other "non-ADHD" disruptive behavior problems, are probably about as common as depression in cases of ADHD and DAMP. In many cases these also culminate around the age of 10, perhaps especially if they are associated with depression, which is common. In other cases the socially acting-out behavior remains through adolescence. In such cases the risk of antisocial development is considerable.

Conduct disorder in a more restrictive sense refers to a deviance in behavior, which leads to suffering of people in the person's environment or to actions that for other reasons are not socially acceptable and would have been deemed "criminal" in older individuals. Aggression, destructiveness toward property and other people (including serious acts of violence), truancy, long and repeated episodes of running away from home during the early school years, starting fires, substance abuse (including taking up smoking cigarettes very early), and acting out sexually at a young age (including promiscuity) are common signs of such a disorder.

Upon starting school, only about one in 10 children with ADHD/DAMP meet the criteria for "conservative" conduct disorder according to the DSM. Three years later, about three to four in 10 do. Just under half of these have a socially acting-out behavior at the age of 13. The majority of this latter group acts out socially in their late teens and young adult years as well and meets the DSM criteria for either antisocial personality disorder or so-called borderline personality disorder. It is especially for this group that there is a great risk of a development toward criminal activity in adult age—if such a career has not already been started.

The correlation between conduct disorder and depression has been mentioned a few times in passing. For these two "endpoint" manifestations of mental ill health to occur simultaneously in ADHD/DAMP so often can seem contradictory. One needs to remember that children have a smaller range of expressions when it comes to mental suffering than adults do. Many depressed children do not perceive themselves as feeling "low," depressed, or even "a bit down." In part this may be because they do not yet have adequate words for their emotions. Their depression is often expressed as irritability, anger, and sadness or being prone to crying, all wrapped into one package, and anger is often expressed through socially unacceptable actions.

It appears as though the prognosis regarding psychosocial adjustment can be somewhat better if conduct disorder in ADHD/DAMP is also associated with depression. This could possibly be explained by the depression itself being a sign of the child developing moral values or, to put it in the words of a different tradition, a superego. Without "morals" the depression might not develop; it is one's own moral values that make one feel bad and worthless. If a child with ADHD/DAMP is acting out socially without depression being involved it may be a manifestation of the moral norms failing, and then it is perhaps not so strange for a socially unacceptable behavior to continue through older years as well. If, on the other hand, there is a set of norms as to what is right and wrong—which, unfortunately, can result in the child with ADHD/DAMP developing depression—there are also favorable conditions for a good or fairly good psychosocial adjustment in adult years.

It is often assumed that the precursor of conduct disorder, ODD (see below), has the same kind of negative outcome overall that is true of "restrictive" conduct disorder. It needs to be pointed out, again and again, that ODD, while being a very common precursor in conduct disorder, *usually* does not lead to conduct disorder. More than half of young children with ODD in the context of ADHD will not go down an antisocial pathway.

In conclusion, it appears as though a very negative psychosocial development in ADHD/DAMP is dependent on the development of conduct disorder/antisocial behavior during the early school years. It is primarily among children with ADHD/DAMP who have also developed antisocial behavior by the age of 10 that there is a great risk of psychosocial maladjustment in adult years. There are, of course, other patients with ADHD/DAMP who also have a negative or uncertain prognosis—for example, the relatively few who develop severe mental illnesses—but more than half of those who do not have an early onset of antisocial behavior seems to manage relatively well in adulthood, at least from the point of view of overall social "adjustment." Academic underachievement, however, may be typical of adult functioning in ADHD, regardless of the presence or not of conduct problems. In a separate chapter, a more thorough description of the prognosis in cases of ADHD/DAMP will be given.

ODD AND PATHOLOGICAL DEMAND AVOIDANCE

Verbal aggression, negativism, saying "no" to most things, and general "defiance" characterize many children with ADHD/DAMP up until puberty (and in some cases thereafter as well). Whether this—with the terminology used in DSM-5—"oppositional defiant disorder" (ODD) should be equated with conduct disorders or as early stages of them is unclear. Many studies indicate that ODD is not closely related to conduct disorder, at least not if conduct disorder is to have such a narrow definition as the one found in the DSM-5. At least half of all the patients with ADHD/DAMP have behaviors that fit under the diagnosis "ODD."

The behavior found in cases of ODD is strongly reminiscent of what one sees in many children of 2 to 4 years of age who get angry, whine, cry, and yell if anything does not go their way or if they simply do not get exactly what they want.

The manifestations of ODD are often worsened in conjunction with feeling particularly low, low self-esteem, and feelings of failure. This can be particularly difficult to distinguish, not least for parents who often spend a great deal of time arguing with the child who "always" opposes everything. To recognize the depressive note in the child's obstinate behavior demands that the parent have a great deal of imagination and manage to stay calm whenever the child is acting out. The flood of swear words that the child pours over the mother, or at worst the teacher, can be followed by gentle crying, and the child's "immaturity" quickly becomes apparent if one can only find the energy to show compassion instead of throwing a tantrum similar to that of the child.

One of the defining symptoms of the DSM category of ODD is "inability to control temper." It is interesting to note that the only symptom shared by (almost) all children with ADHD is the inability to control emotions (Kadesjö, C., et al., 2003). It remains unclear to what extent emotional lability is actually part and parcel of the "ADHD syndrome" itself and not an indication of a separate oppositional disorder. Emotional lability may well be closely linked to overall executive dysfunction in ADHD/ODD (McKay and Halperin 2001).

A group of children presents with a rather peculiar type of oppositional behaviors, sometimes now subsumed under the label of "pathological demand avoidance" syndrome (PDA). Boys and girls with PDA will do anything to avoid meeting the demands of adults and children alike. The behaviors "used" in maintaining avoidance range from openly oppositional or manipulative to "extreme shyness," passivity, and muteness. PDA has been suggested to be a variant of an autism spectrum condition, but it is as likely that any kind of ESSENCE, including language disorder and ADHD, could be the underlying problem in PDA.

DRUG AND OTHER SUBSTANCE ABUSE

Substance abuse, which is sometimes defined as belonging in the diagnostic category of conduct disorder, is relatively common in ADHD/DAMP, at least in the late teens and young adult years (Wilens & Morrison, 2011). It is often a case of early onset of alcohol use, and exaggerated use at that; more rarely is it a question of heavy (isolated) abuse of a different kind. Nicotine use is also much more common, is more intense, and has an earlier life start in ADHD than in perhaps any other group in modern Western societies.

It is possible that "pathological intoxication"(i.e., a disproportionately strong reaction even to small amounts of alcohol) is more common among people with ADHD/DAMP than among the population at large, but there is a lack of conclusive studies on this subject. It is important to "warn" parents of children with ADHD, teenagers with the disorder, and adults who are diagnosed later in life that pathological reactions to alcohol (and possibly also other drugs, including benzodiazepines) can happen and lead to devastating consequences.

There is a very large—and growing—body of evidence to suggest that the rate of ADHD/DAMP (and other ESSENCE) among adults with different types of addictions is extremely high: perhaps one third to two thirds of all severe alcohol and drug abusers have such a background. The strong relationship between severe drug abuse (including chronic alcoholism, amphetamine, "grass," and cocaine dependence) and ADHD/DAMP/ESSENCE needs to be noted by adult psychiatrists, general practitioners, nurses, education specialists, and social workers so that underlying problems might be intervened for in an appropriate way. Recent studies suggest a strongly beneficial effect of treatment for ADHD on the outcome for young male violent offenders in prisons (with diagnosed ADHD), to mention just one area in which a better understanding of the correlation between ADHD and substance abuse (and, in the longer-term perspective, criminal acts) will lead to important changes in practice in many adult services/institutions.

DIFFICULTIES IN SOCIAL INTERACTION—AUTISTIC TRAITS AND ASPERGER SYNDROME

A large percentage of children with severe ADHD/DAMP and other ESSENCE have difficulties interacting with other children in a frictionless manner. At least three out of four have problems with peers in different ways. Every other child with severe DAMP in addition has many other symptoms reminiscent of those found in autism, for example stereotypic movements and grammatical and pragmatic difficulties in language. For many of these people, the description "autistic traits" or "autism spectrum disorder"/"autistic-like condition" may be called for. In other cases, it can be difficult to differentiate from the typical presentation of Asperger syndrome. Nevertheless, it should be pointed out that even children with severe DAMP can possess exceptional empathetic ability and be far removed from the autism spectrum.

Even children with mild and moderate DAMP often have problems relating to peers. In the Gothenburg study of DAMP in the 1970s it turned out that 60% to 70% of 6- to 7-year-olds with milder forms of DAMP had such great difficulties interacting with other children that they generally were not included in other children's games. Yet when meeting them one could determine that their difficulties in interaction were not equally inhibiting as the ones found in autism. It was not, to the same extent, a question of lacking or having significantly lowered empathy; it seemed to be more of a matter of problems in concentration and attention that made it difficult to perceive other people's reactions quickly enough. Impulsiveness and hyperactivity could also bring about actions that other children could not understand or accept, which in turn led to them reacting by becoming angry with or ostracizing the child with DAMP.

In the Gothenburg study, four out of 10 subjects in their late teens with DAMP were described as socially negative or avoidant. Many of these had a social phobia and avoided social situations if possible. They also stated that they often felt down, and just under half met the criteria for depression (or, in a few cases, for manic depressive/bipolar disorder). Some were significantly handicapped by their social phobia even though they were ostensibly "well adjusted." Almost one in 10 in the peer group without DAMP had similar social negativity or socially avoidant behavior.

TICS AND TOURETTE SYNDROME

It is still unknown how many people with ADHD/DAMP have tics, motor or phonic. Motor tics are very common within the general population; at least one in 10 children have, for some period of time, between the age of 5 and 12 had spasmodic motor movements of different kinds, including shaking one's head "to get one's hair out of one's eyes," blinking one's eyes, and twitches in one's shoulders or the corners of one's lips. Many also carry on with obsessive-compulsive sounds, for example clearing their throats, blowing their noses, and whistling. These kinds of sounds are sometimes referred to as phonic tics.

It is known that many children with severe tics—and particularly those with Tourette syndrome (i.e., the combination of motor tics and phonic tics)—have attention deficit, hyperactivity, and impulsiveness. Many, in some studies more than half, meet the criteria for ADHD and DAMP.

SLEEP DISORDERS

Almost half of all children and adolescents with ADHD have sleep problems or suffer from sleep disorders (Miano et al., 2012). Five different sleep patterns/styles have been proposed in ADHD: (i) a sleep pattern characterized mainly by a hypo-arousal state, resembling severe hypersomnia and/or narcolepsy, which may be considered a "primary" form of ADHD (i.e., without the interference of other sleep disorders); (ii) a pattern associated with delayed sleep-onset latency and with—possibly—a higher risk of bipolar disorder; (iii) one associated with sleep-disordered breathing; (iv) another related to restless legs syndrome and/or periodic limb movements; and (v) lastly, a phenotype related to epilepsy/or EEG interictal discharges. Each of the five sleep patterns is characterized by specific sleep alterations expressed by either increased or decreased levels of arousal during sleep, and these may have important treatment implications. Treatment with stimulants can be recommended perhaps particularly in the "primary" form of ADHD, whereas treatment of the main sleep disorders or of comorbidities (i.e., bipolar disorders and epilepsy) might be the preferred intervention in the other four sleep phenotypes. The sleep phenotypes (ii), (iii), and (iv) appear to be associated with an increased level of arousal during sleep. Some studies have suggested that both an increase and a decrease in arousal can be accounted for by executive dysfunctions controlled by prefrontal cortical regions (the main cortical areas implicated in the pathogenesis of ADHD) and by primary dysfunction in the arousal system, which may be hyperactivated or hypoactivated depending on the form of ADHD/sleep phenotype.

EATING DISORDERS (INCLUDING ANOREXIA, BULIMIA, AND OVERWEIGHT)

A number of retrospective studies have shown ADHD to be a common problem in chronic eating disorders, including anorexia nervosa and bulimia nervosa (Wentz et al., 2005). Both retrospective and prospective studies have indicated a (relatively strong) link between ADHD and obesity (Hölcke et al., 2008; Shaw et al., 2012). A rather common vicious circle in children with inattentive ADHD and DAMP is one in which the child is excluded early on from all kinds of physical activity (including PE at school, either as a result of bullying or as a self-chosen phenomenon) and gradual overeating or multi-impulsive behaviors lead to either bulimia or obesity. Interesting preliminary studies of stimulant treatment for children and adolescents with severe obesity and "comorbid" ADHD indicate that such intervention might be effective in reducing overweight dramatically in affected individuals (Dahlgren, 2012 [personal communication]).

"SEVERE" MENTAL DISORDERS—SCHIZOPHRENIA AND MANIC-DEPRESSIVE ILLNESS ("BIPOLAR DISORDER")

Older follow-up studies of "MBD" often depicted a negative outlook with a very high risk of severe mental disorder. This has been revised, and it now seems to be a question of only a relatively small group who develop, for example, schizophrenia or manic-depressive (bipolar) disorder. Given the fact that as of yet children with DAMP/ESSENCE have been followed up only to about age 35 and that most studies on ADHD do not even extend that far, it is, however, too soon to draw any definitive conclusions.

In the Gothenburg study of ADHD with DCD (=DAMP), a relatively high proportion of people developed manic-depressive disorder in their late teens. No one in the peer group without ADHD had been diagnosed in the same manner. Earlier studies had indicated that at most 0.2% of the entire population of that age group would have received such a diagnosis. No one in the Gothenburg study had developed schizophrenia. At age 22, however, one individual in the DAMP group had symptoms that corresponded to a "schizophrenia spectrum" disorder (including schizoid and schizotypal personality disorder). That said, it is still too early to tell whether this really represents an increased risk of schizophrenia, or if it is merely a random statistical correlation. Manic-depressive disorder (bipolar disorder) with very early onset (before 5 years of age) is rare but can easily be confused, or appear together, with ADHD/DAMP. Extreme hyperactivity, impulsiveness, irritability, aggressiveness, and violent mood swings in small children should be examined with bipolar disorder as a possible explanation, especially if there is a genetic predisposition for it in the family.

MISCELLANEOUS

There is, as of yet, no convincing evidence that different types of psychosomatic symptoms, for example stomachache and headache, have anything to do with ADHD or DAMP problems (Almog et al., 2010). The same seems to go for mental symptoms and disorders dominated by anxiety (even though, as already mentioned, the core symptoms of ADHD may sometimes be "over interpreted" as anxiety disorder). All manner of adult psychiatric problems can have been preceded by ADHD/DAMP problems during childhood. In some studies of young adults with mental disorders it has turned out that problems with DAMP have been significantly more prevalent than expected. This has been the case in, for example, adolescents with psychoses. Since the terms "ADHD" and "DAMP" are relatively unknown within adult psychiatry it is common for DAMP problems to go unnoticed there. A recent study from the south of Sweden suggested that one in five to one in four of *all* adult psychiatric outpatients actually have ADHD, but only a tiny proportion of these have actually received a diagnosis of ADHD.

Apart from the conditions that have already been mentioned, it is very common in cases of ADHD/DAMP to find symptoms that can be perceived as signs of different types of personality disorders. Borderline/personality disorder is often stated to have had "MBD precursors" of different kinds. The Gothenburg study, however, showed only a weak correlation between showing signs of borderline personality as a teenager and being diagnosed with DAMP as a child. The reverse conditions apply for adults, though: among adult psychiatric patients diagnosed with personality disorder, the majority have a history of ADHD/DAMP and/or autism spectrum disorder. Also, there is emerging evidence that hyperactivity in childhood/adolescence may be a marker for later chronic pain syndrome, fibromyalgia, and various types of fatigue syndromes. There is a great need for further follow-up studies of the populations of children with ADHD/ DAMP who have been examined in early childhood and who are now in their thirties, forties, and fifties.

CONCLUDING REMARKS

ADHD/DAMP should be seen as a deviation from normal psychomotor development that does not, however, inevitably bring about psychiatric problems. Psychiatric problems of different kinds, including depression, anxiety, conduct disorder, tics, and autistic traits, are nevertheless very common. Doctors and psychologists who are responsible for adequate measures being implemented in ADHD/DAMP and other ESSENCE must be well versed in the additional psychiatric problems brought on by or associated with the underlying condition in order to be able to suggest appropriate treatment. Also, doctors, child and adult specialists alike, need to be upto date and experienced in ADHD/DAMP when dealing with people with mental health problems of any type. ADHD/DAMP and other ESSENCE are clearly extremely common underlying conditions in a wide variety of mental health disorders, ranging from conduct and oppositional disorders, to depression and anxiety, through to personality disorder, substance abuse, and criminality.

REFERENCES

Almog, M., Gabis, L.V., Shefer, S., & Bujanover, Y. (2010). [Gastrointestinal symptoms in pediatric patients with attention deficit and hyperactivity disorders]. *Harefuah, 149*, 33–36, 62.

Bramham, J., Murphy, D.G., Xenitidis, K., Asherson, P., Hopkin, G., & Young, S. (2012). Adults with attention deficit hyperactivity disorder: an investigation of age-related differences in behavioural symptoms, neuropsychological function and co-morbidity. *Psychological Medicine, 42*, 2225–2234.

Gillberg, I.C., & Gillberg, C. (1989). Children with preschool minor neurodevelopmental disorders. IV: Behaviour and school achievement at age 13. *Developmental Medicine and Child Neurology, 31*, 3–13.

Hellgren, L., Gillberg, I.C., Bågenholm, A., & Gillberg, C. (1994). Children with deficits in attention, motor control and perception (DAMP) almost grown up: psychiatric and personality disorders at age 16 years. *Journal of Child Psychology and Psychiatry, 35*, 1255–1271.

Hinshaw, S.P., Owens, E.B., Zalecki, C., Huggins, S.P., Montenegro-Nevado, A.J., Schrodek, E., et al. (2012). Prospective follow-up of girls with attention-deficit/hyperactivity disorder into early adulthood: Continuing impairment includes elevated risk for suicide attempts and self-injury. *Journal of Consulting and Clinical Psychology, 80*, 1041–1051.

Hölcke, M., Marcus, C., Gillberg, C., & Fernell, E. (2008). Paediatric obesity: a neurodevelopmental perspective. *Acta Paediatrica, 97*, 819–821.

Kadesjö, C., Hagglöf, B., Kadesjö, B., & Gillberg, C. (2003). Attention-deficit-hyperactivity disorder with and without oppositional defiant disorder in 3- to 7-year-old children. *Developmental Medicine and Child Neurology, 45*, 693–699.

McCarthy, S., Cranswick, N., Potts, L., Taylor, E., & Wong, I.C. (2009). Mortality associated with attention-deficit hyperactivity disorder (ADHD) drug treatment: a retrospective cohort study of children, adolescents and young adults using the general practice research database. *Drug Safety, 32*, 1089–1096.

McKay, K.E., & Halperin, J.M. (2001) ADHD, aggression, and antisocial behavior across the lifespan. Interactions with neurochemical and cognitive function. *Annals of the New York Academy of Sciences, 931*, 84–96.

Miano, S., Parisi, P., Villa, M.P. (2012). The sleep phenotypes of attention deficit hyperactivity disorder: the role of arousal during sleep and implications for treatment. *Medical Hypotheses, 79*, 147–153.

Shaw, M., Hodgkins, P., Caci, H., Young, S., Kahle, J., Woods, A.G., et al. (2012). A systematic review and analysis of long-term outcomes in attention deficit hyperactivity disorder: effects of treatment and non-treatment. *BMC Medicine, 10*, 99.

Simon, V., Czobor, P., & Bitter, I. (2013). Is ADHD severity in adults associated with the lifetime prevalence of comorbid depressive episodes and anxiety disorders? *European Psychiatry, 28*(5), 308–314.

Thapar, A., Cooper, M., Jefferies, R., & Stergiakouli, E. (2012). What causes attention deficit hyperactivity disorder? *Archives of Disease in Childhood, 97*, 260–265.

Wilens, T.E., & Morrison, N.R. (2011). The intersection of attention-deficit/hyperactivity disorder and substance abuse. *Current Opinion in Psychiatry, 24*, 280–285.

Wentz, E., Lacey, J.H., Waller, G., Råstam, M., Turk, J., & Gillberg, C. (2005). Childhood onset neuropsychiatric disorders in adult eating disorder patients. A pilot study. *European Child & Adolescent Psychiatry, 14*, 431–437.

Other Associated Problems Not Classified as Mental or Psychiatric Disorders

ADHD/DAMP and other ESSENCE either grant a predisposition to, or may for other reasons be associated with a variety of problems (or non-problem characteristics that are not typical of the general population) that do not fall within the definition of ADHD/DAMP/ ESSENCE itself and that cannot be classified as mental or psychiatric disorders. Among these are non-right-handedness, sleep problems, febrile seizures, and accidents or near-accidents. A number of other factors/problems have occasionally been stated to be associated with ADHD/DAMP, but convincing proof of this correlation has not been brought forth. Among these are allergies and autoimmunity (allergic reactions to one's own body).

LEFT-HANDEDNESS AND AMBIDEXTERITY

ADHD/DAMP and other ESSENCE are, in quite a number of cases, associated with ambidexterity, and in others still with left-handedness (Rodriguez & Waldenström, 2008). It is, however, questionable whether this should be classified as a problem. The rate of children who are not clearly right-handed is significantly increased in cases of ESSENCE. The reasons for the correlation are unclear. Slow development of the nervous system is one possibility; younger children are more often ambidextrous. Brain damage is another explanation; the rate of left-handedness is always relatively high in a group of people with damage in either cerebral hemisphere (Bishop, 1980; Gillberg et al., 1984). Certain hereditary factors and intrauterine stress are probably also important in certain cases. It is also entirely possible that two or more of the suggested causes work together in individual cases.

In cases of ADHD without DCD, there is no consistent evidence of increased rates of non-right-handedness. However, there is ample support for the view that there is abnormal brain laterality from neuropsychological, EEG, MRI, fMRI, and diffusion tensor imaging studies (Dramsdahl et al., 2012; Gillberg, 2010; Gilliam et al., 2011). Nevertheless, it is unclear what this means, both in terms of pathogenesis and when it comes to possible clinical implications.

SLEEP PROBLEMS AND OTHER DEVIANCIES IN SLEEP PATTERNS

The group of children with ADHD/DAMP and other ESSENCE who have early onset of hyperactivity often have an irregular sleep rhythm, with frequent awakenings during the night, and many require comparatively little sleep during their first several years of life (Scott et al., 2013; Voinescu et al., 2012). These problems can continue throughout their entire childhood but sometimes develop into a normal sleep pattern or even something that appears to be an increased need for sleep (Kirov et al., 2012). During their school years it is common for children with ADHD/DAMP/ ESSENCE to be extremely tired upon arriving home in the afternoon and they may need to sleep for an hour, sometimes more, to have the energy for any other activity during the rest of the day.

Many people with ADHD have difficulty unwinding in the evenings and tend to stay up late at night. As a consequence they are often tired

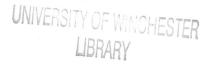

in the morning. Generally speaking, it is common among people with ADHD/DAMP to have a special circadian rhythm: morning fatigue with crankiness, irritability, and low alertness during the morning hours, often combined with hyperactivity and generally disruptive behavior, increasing alertness and possibly good ability to concentrate, during the early afternoon hours, and thereafter a slump in alertness with fatigue, hyperactivity, or sleep in the late afternoon and then maximum alertness and relatively good ability to concentrate in the evening and later hours. Some individuals with ADHD are so tired during the early parts of the day as to qualify for a diagnosis of chronic fatigue syndrome (Sáez-Francàs et al., 2012).

Many individuals with ADHD have hypersomnia, and a small group show all the symptoms of narcolepsy (Miano et al., 2012). There are also occasional cases of the so-called Kleine-Levin syndrome (episodic hypersomnia with episodic hyperphagia) associated with ADHD and other symptoms common in ESSENCE. The co-occurrence of ADHD-type problems, Kleine-Levin syndrome, and PANDAS has been described in an 11-year-old girl (Das & Radhakrishnan, 2012).

It is not uncommon for people with ADHD/DAMP to make annoying sounds upon falling asleep or while sleeping, during periods of deeper sleep. Moving one's entire body and rolling or banging one's head are also relatively common.

Nightmares and night terrors (i.e., a nocturnal state of confusion in conjunction with obstructed breathing such as in cases of snoring, nasal congestion, or "adenoids") are common in ADHD (Silvestri et al., 2009), but it is still unclear whether they are *particularly* common in cases of ADHD/DAMP. However, from a purely theoretical standpoint, it is likely that weak muscle tone/hypotonia and an aberrant state of wakefulness in the nervous system could predispose to this type of problem, perhaps especially for night terrors. Also, long-term clinical experience does suggest a relatively strong link between ADHD and night terrors.

There are also individuals with ADHD who show a type of rhythmic movement disorder (headbanging, legbanging, body rocking) during non-REM stage 2 sleep (with EEG K-complexes), and this can cause much parental concern. They are benign, however, and affected individuals are amnesic in the morning (Dyken et al., 1997).

The restless legs syndrome is probably also strongly overrepresented in individuals with ADHD (Gagliano et al., 2011). It is quite common for children with ADHD who have night terrors to also have rhythmic movement disorder as previously described and restless legs syndrome.

Some children with ADHD/DAMP/ESSENCE are sleepwalkers and talk a lot in their sleep (Silvestri et al., 2009), but it is uncertain in these cases as well whether there really is any connection to the ADHD/DAMP problems as such. For a small but not negligible group of children with ADHD/DAMP, there are problems with sudden onset of and generally "non-negotiable" need for sleep. The transition from being awake to a state of deep sleep can take only a few seconds. In these instances the case is sometimes narcolepsy—that is, involuntary sleep, often in combination with total loss of muscle tone and sometimes also with a special type of hallucinations upon falling asleep. In those, rare, patients with ADHD/DAMP and narcolepsy, treatment with stimulant medications is generally called for. In other cases, the diagnostic criteria for narcolepsy are not met, but the hypersomnia might be disabling just the same. Milder stimulants (including caffeine) can be helpful in such cases.

EPILEPSY, INCLUDING FEBRILE SEIZURES

In the Gothenburg ADHD/DAMP study there was a much increased prevalence of febrile seizures in the DAMP group relative to controls (Rasmussen et al., 1983). Since such a correlation has not yet been demonstrated in other studies, definite conclusions regarding a connection between DAMP and a lowered seizure threshold have to await replication studies. If the correlation is "real" it is possible that immaturity in the central nervous system leads both to a lowered seizure threshold with subsequent increased risk of febrile seizures and to symptoms consistent with a DAMP diagnosis. It is unlikely that the febrile seizures themselves would be the cause of DAMP.

Epilepsy (febrile seizures not included) is *not* very common in cases of ADHD or DAMP. Nevertheless, there could still be a strong correlation between epilepsy and ADHD/DAMP, as indicated by a number of studies on ADHD and by a number of studies on epilepsy (e.g., Cohen et al., 2013; Neville, 2013). More large-scale studies of children with epilepsy with particular emphasis on ADHD/DAMP are needed to shed further light on this matter. A few recent studies do suggest that children with seizures are at much increased risk of attention deficits (McLellan et al., 2005; Reilly et al., 2013) and perhaps a somewhat increased proclivity for hyperactivity. Some of these children do meet the criteria for ADHD/ DAMP, even though the majority probably do not. In patients with the combination of IDD and epilepsy, hyperactivity and difficulties in concentration are very common, but it remains uncertain whether epilepsy without IDD is also associated with this type of problem. In cases of temporal lobe/psychomotor epilepsy (complex partial seizures), the rate of ADHD and similar problems is significantly increased, but in such cases it is also uncertain whether children of average or above-average intelligence are at any greater risk.

MEMORY PROBLEMS

Attention deficit, difficulties in concentration, and lacking a sense of time are common symptoms in cases of ADHD/DAMP (Noreika et al., 2013; Nydén et al., 2000). It would not be unexpected if such difficulties would give the impression that there might be problems with the person's memory. It is also debatable to what extent difficulties in memory can be entirely separated from problems in concentration and attention. Boys with ADHD show impaired information storage (Rhodes et al., 2012). Interestingly, boys with ADHD plus ODD have an even more pronounced problem in this respect. Many researchers view the "working memory" or the "short-term memory" as being intimately linked with certain attention functions. The difficulties in automation, which are so accentuated in cases of DAMP, also create problems with actively mobilizing memory functions.

It is well known from clinical experience that children with ADHD/ DAMP and adults who have been diagnosed with ADHD/DAMP/ MBD since childhood have special difficulties in mobilizing names and words, and also have timing deficits in this respect (Noreika et al., 2013). "Dysnomia" is a technical term that is used to describe the specific difficulty in quickly remembering or producing names of people and places that one knows are actually firmly imprinted. Problems in general with mobilizing "the correct word," for example during conversation with many quick shifts and turns, are very common and are mirrored in utterances such as, "what's the word" and "I mean, uh, I mean...." The disorder can, in this respect, occasionally be so severe that it can be reasonable to consider the diagnosis of dysphasia (a milder degree of aphasia).

These problems with quickly accessing information often lead to frustration from people who do not understand what ADHD/DAMP means—and sometimes even from those who do understand. One might wonder about things such as the knowledge having been there the day before, but now appearing to have vanished. Or one feels convinced that if the child simply tried a little harder, if he or she just focused, things would go better—"I think he probably could do it if he would just put his mind to it!"

There can also be problems with long-term memory, even if these are rarely equally accentuated as the aforementioned "difficulties in mobilization."

ACCIDENTS

Children with hyperactivity and ADHD/DAMP are at a much greater risk of ending up in both trivial and serious accidents than other children (including the non-ADHD siblings of children with ADHD) (Shilon et al., 2012). Yet one could argue that many seem to have luck on their side; the majority manage to avoid any serious accidents or injuries up to adulthood and beyond. Facial, skull, arm, and leg fractures occur up to five times as often in children with ADHD/DAMP as they do in children without such a diagnosis. Their bruises are more numerous and more widespread than those of other children. This sometimes leads to suspicion that the child is being subjected to abuse, which is generally not the case. On the other hand, children with ADHD/DAMP are hyperactive, have difficulty concentrating, often have both ODD and conduct disorder as well, and are not rarely so exasperating that they run a greater risk of being subjected to physical punishment/abuse. It can therefore among other things be very difficult to determine causality in cases of ADHD/DAMP where child abuse is suspected.

Road traffic accidents are strongly associated with disruptive behavior disorders, including ADHD, in young males (Redelmeier et al., 2010). A broad review of the scientific literature demonstrated well-documented driving risks and impairments associated with ADHD, and positive effects of stimulant medications on driving performance (Barkley & Cox, 2007). Children with ADHD/DAMP run out into the street in the middle of traffic much more often than others (Stavrinos et al., 2011) and occasionally run their bike into walls, cars, and other people. They often fall into the water or down from roofs or trees, and hence they naturally put themselves at great risk of encountering accidents. The most surprising aspect is actually really the fact that there are not even more serious accidents and that the outcome, in spite of the injuries and fractures that do occur, is still—almost always—relatively happy.

It is not uncommon for children with ADHD/DAMP to ingest detergents or solvents, medicines, or alcoholic beverages even during their preschool years. Children without ADHD/DAMP can also try these types of things but generally stop themselves quickly, for example because they encounter a consistency or taste that they are not familiar with.

MISCELLANEOUS

ADHD/DAMP has long been stated to be associated with allergy and autoimmune disease, a correlation that, in addition, could possibly be associated with left-handedness and the effects of testosterone on the developing nervous system. As of yet there is no empirical evidence supporting a specific correlation between ADHD/DAMP and allergy/autoimmunity

(Martino et al., 2009; Schmitt et al., 2010). Allergy is extremely common within the population at large, and it does not seem to be even more common among children with ADHD/DAMP. This does not mean that certain children with ADHD/DAMP and allergy could constitute a subgroup that could be in need of special attention, for example in conjunction with arranging a treatment program (see separate chapter on interventions). Children with eczema appear to have an increased rate of ADHD, but the mechanisms of the association are not understood.

Enuresis is considerable more common in children and adolescents with ADHD than those without the disorder (Mellon et al., 2013). A similar trend is seen in respect of encopresis.

CONCLUDING REMARKS

ADHD/DAMP occurs together with other conditions and problems outlined in this chapter, including sleep problems and febrile seizures/epilepsy. Ambidexterity and left-handedness are relatively common. Many children with ADHD/DAMP are prone to accidents. It is important for clinicians and parents to be aware of these (sometimes very strong) correlations so that all children with ADHD/DAMP can receive appropriate help, not just for one aspect of their problems but for all of them.

REFERENCES

Barkley, R.A., & Cox, D. (2007). A review of driving risks and impairments associated with attention-deficit/hyperactivity disorder and the effects of stimulant medication on driving performance. *Journal of Safety Research, 38*, 113–128.

Bishop, D. V. (1980). Handedness, clumsiness and cognitive ability. *Developmental Medicine and Child Neurology, 22*, 569–579.

Cohen, R., Senecky, Y., Shuper, A., Inbar, D., Chodick, G., Shalev, V., et al. (2013). Prevalence of epilepsy and attention-deficit hyperactivity (ADHD) disorder: a population-based study. *Journal of Child Neurology, 28*, 120–123.

Das, A., & Radhakrishnan, A. (2012). A case of PANDAS with Kleine-Levin type periodic hypersomnia. *Sleep Medicine, 13*, 319–320.

Dramsdahl, M., Westerhausen, R., Haavik, J., Hugdahl, K., & Plessen, K.J. (2012). Adults with attention-deficit/hyperactivity disorder—a diffusion-tensor imaging study of the corpus callosum. *Psychiatry Research, 201*, 168–173.

Dyken, M.E., Lin-Dyken, D.C., & Yamada, T. (1997). Diagnosing rhythmic movement disorder with video-polysomnography. *Pediatric Neurology, 16*, 37–41.

Gagliano, A., Aricò, I., Calarese, T., Condurso, R., Germanò, E., Cedro, C., et al. (2011). Restless Leg Syndrome in ADHD children: levetiracetam as a reasonable therapeutic option. *Brain & Development, 33*, 480–486.

Gillberg, C. (2010). The ESSENCE in child psychiatry: early symptomatic syndromes eliciting neurodevelopmental clinical examinations. *Research in Developmental Disabilities, 31*, 1543–1551.

Gillberg, C., Waldenström, E., & Rasmussen, P. (1984). Handedness in Swedish 10-year-olds. Some background and associated factors. *Journal of Child Psychology and Psychiatry, 25*, 421–432.

Gilliam, M., Stockman, M., Malek, M., Sharp, W., Greenstein, D., Lalonde, F., et al. (2011). Developmental trajectories of the corpus callosum in attention-deficit/hyperactivity disorder. *Biological Psychiatry, 69*, 839–846.

Kirov, R., Uebel, H., Albrecht, B., Banaschewski, T., Yordanova, J., & Rothenberger, A. (2012). Attention-deficit/hyperactivity disorder (ADHD) and adaptation night as determinants of sleep patterns in children. *European Child & Adolescent Psychiatry, 21*, 681–690.

Martino, D., Defazio, G., & Giovannoni, G. (2009). The PANDAS subgroup of tic disorders and childhood-onset obsessive-compulsive disorder. *Journal of Psychosomatic Research, 67*, 547–557.

McLellan, A., Davies, S., Heyman, I., Harding, B., Harkness, W., Taylor, D., et al. (2005). Psychopathology in children with epilepsy before and after temporal lobe resection. *Developmental Medicine and Child Neurology, 47*, 666–672.

Mellon, M.W., Natchev, B.E., Katusic, S.K., Colligan, R.C., Weaver, A.L., Voigt, R.G. et al. (2013) Incidence of enuresis and encopresis among children with attention-deficit/ hyperactivity disorder in a population-based birth cohort. *Academic Pediatrics, 13*, 322–327.

Miano, S., Parisi, P., & Villa, M.P. (2012). The sleep phenotypes of attention deficit hyperactivity disorder: the role of arousal during sleep and implications for treatment. *Medical Hypotheses, 79*, 147–153.

Neville, B. (2013). Role of ESSENCE for preschool children with neurodevelopmental disorders. *Brain & Development, 35*(2), 128–132.

Noreika, V., Falter, C.M., & Rubia, K. (2013) Timing deficits in attention-deficit/hyperactivity disorder (ADHD): Evidence from neurocognitive and neuroimaging studies. *Neuropsychologia, 51*(2), 235–266.

Nydén, A., Hjelmquist, E., & Gillberg, C. (2000). Autism spectrum and attention-deficit disorders in girls. Some neuropsychological aspects. *European Child and Adolescent Psychiatry, 9*, 180–185.

Rasmussen, P., Gillberg, C., Waldenström, E., & Svenson, B. (1983). Perceptual, motor and attentional deficits in seven-year-old children: neurological and neurodevelopmental aspects. *Developmental Medicine and Child Neurology, 25*, 315–333.

Redelmeier, D.A., Chan, W.K., & Lu, H. (2010). Road trauma in teenage male youth with childhood disruptive behavior disorders: a population based analysis. *PLoS Medicine, 7*, e1000369.

Reilly, C., Atkinson, P., Gillberg, C., Scott, R., DasK., Chin, R., Aylett, S., Burch, V., & Neville, B. (2013). *The identification of educational problems of children with epilepsy. Poster Presentation.* British Paediatric Neurology Association Annual Conference, Manchester, UK, January 23–25, 2013.

Rhodes, S.M., Park, J., Seth, S., & Coghill, D.R. (2012). A comprehensive investigation of memory impairment in attention deficit hyperactivity disorder and oppositional defiant disorder. *Journal of Child Psychology and Psychiatry, 53*, 128–137.

Rodriguez, A., & Waldenström, U. (2008). Fetal origins of child non-right-handedness and mental health. *Journal of Child Psychology and Psychiatry, 49*, 967–976.

Sáez-Francàs, N., Alegre, J., Calvo, N., Antonio Ramos-Quiroga, J., Ruiz, E., Hernández-Vara, J., et al. (2012). Attention-deficit hyperactivity disorder in chronic fatigue syndrome patients. *Psychiatry Research, 200*, 748–753.

Schmitt, J., Buske-Kirschbaum, A., & Roessner, V. (2010). Is a topic disease a risk factor for attention-deficit/hyperactivity disorder? A systematic review. *Allergy, 65*, 1506–1524.

Scott, N., Blair, P.S., Emond, A.M., Fleming, P.J., Humphreys, J.S., Henderson, J., et al. (2013). Sleep patterns in children with ADHD: a population-based cohort study from birth to 11 years. *Journal of Sleep Research, 22*(2), 121–128.

Shilon, Y., Pollak, Y., Aran, A., Shaked, S., & Gross-Tsur, V. (2012). Accidental injuries are more common in children with attention deficit hyperactivity disorder compared with their non-affected siblings. *Child: Care, Health and Development, 38*, 366–370.

Silvestri, R., Gagliano, A., Aricò, I., Calarese, T., Cedro, C., Bruni, O., et al. (2009). Sleep disorders in children with attention-deficit/hyperactivity disorder (ADHD) recorded overnight by video-polysomnography. *Sleep Medicine, 10*, 1132–1138.

Stavrinos, D., Biasini, F.J., Fine, P.R., Hodgens, J.B., Khatri, S., Mrug, S., et al. (2011). Mediating factors associated with pedestrian injury in children with attention-deficit/hyperactivity disorder. *Pediatrics, 128*, 296–302.

Voinescu, B.I., Szentagotai, A., & David, D. (2012). Sleep disturbance, circadian preference and symptoms of adult attention deficit hyperactivity disorder (ADHD). *Journal of Neural Transmission, 119*, 1195–1204.

Differentiation from Other Conditions—Differential Diagnosis

ADHD/DAMP and other ESSENCE are, in and of themselves, a heterogeneous set of problems and probably entail a number of more distinct syndromes, even though we do not always have adequate information to tell these apart from each other (Gillberg, 2010; Neville, 2013). At the same time, it should also be said that ADHD represents a set of problems that are fairly similar in nature across cases. Clearly, the aim for us in the future is to be able to diagnose more precisely which brain function disorders that give rise to ADHD/DAMP and other ESSENCE, and when that happens we will probably also have other names for the varying clinical expressions. However, that point still seems far off, and we are referred to the relatively rough ESSENCE categories that currently exist.

ADHD/DAMP overlaps a number of other clinical diagnoses. This is basically not a question of anything more remarkable than disorders in the brain not exactly respecting the behavioral delimitations outlined in, for example, the DSM.

It can sometimes be difficult to determine whether ADHD/DAMP overlaps another condition, such as dyslexia, or if dyslexia itself is the relevant "main" diagnosis and the ADHD/DAMP problems are minimal or nonexistent. This kind of distinction is sometimes crucial, not least when one has to decide whether a child belongs to a group with certain legal rights, for example children with IDD or ASD, or if certain examinations are called for or not, for example when there is suspicion of specific neurological or genetic disorders.

This chapter gives an overview of the most important conditions and disorders that can cause problems of differential diagnosis in cases of ADHD/DAMP.

DIFFICULTIES IN READING AND WRITING

Many parts of this book have addressed the fact that difficulties in reading and writing are common among people with ADHD/DAMP and other ESSENCE. It is commonly the case that issues are raised over whether a child has ADHD *or*, for instance, dyslexia. Questions of this kind are made more difficult by the limits of both ADHD/DAMP and dyslexia not being entirely clear.

A large proportion of people with ADHD have pronounced problems with reading and writing, at least during their first years of school. About half of these have the "specific" form of difficulties in reading and writing known as dyslexia—that is, difficulties that are disproportionate to the individual's general intelligence level.

Judging from population rates of ADHD/DAMP and dyslexia one would have to assume that a quarter to a half of all people with dyslexia also have ADHD/DAMP. It is also common for children with other types of difficulties in reading and writing to have DAMP.

These facts amount to the following:

1. A minority of children with ADHD/DAMP do not develop any kind of difficulties in reading and writing.
2. Approximately every other child with dyslexia does not have ADHD or DCD or both (=DAMP).
3. A majority of all children with difficulties in reading and writing do not have ADHD or DCD.

Despite what has been said, it is uncommon for children and adolescents with dyslexia to not have *any symptom* of ADHD, even if there are not sufficient difficulties to warrant an ADHD diagnosis. Problems with concentration and attention are particularly frequent. It can, however, be difficult to determine which set of problems should be regarded as the primary one; the difficulties in concentration or the dyslexia. If a "real" ADHD/DAMP problem has existed since early childhood it is fair to consider it as primary or at least chronologically preceding the dyslexia. On the other hand, it is hard not to imagine that dyslexia can lead to difficulties in concentration, at least those that appear primarily while reading; how is one supposed to manage to maintain complete concentration if one realizes that one will not be able to complete a task?

To determine whether the difficulties in reading and writing are isolated or associated with ADHD/DAMP, medical examination, psychological evaluation, and reading and writing tests are needed. Because ADHD/DAMP and other ESSENCE are so common among children with dyslexia and other types of difficulties in reading and writing, and the fact that difficulties in reading and writing are so common in cases of ESSENCE generally, all of these examinations need to be performed if suspicion of either diagnosis arises.

IDD

One in seven to one in five of all children with ADHD/DAMP function intellectually at about the same level as found in "special schools" or "classrooms for the educationally subnormal." This means that their IQ is around or below 70. In some of these cases it is truly a question of general borderline intelligence or IDD. However, in many cases, a few subtests from the psychological assessment weigh down the overall result so much that the child functions on par with children in "special schools," even though the results on most of the other subtests suggest that he or she has a normal "baseline intelligence."

If it is clear from the start that the child has IDD, often neither a DCD nor an ADHD diagnosis is given. This is sometimes a reasonable approach within research but can lead to significant problems in clinical practice. Some children suffering from mild, moderate, and severe IDD have so many problems with attention, motor control, and perception that the impression of ADHD/DAMP is striking. If the difficulties cannot easily be explained by a combination of the borderline level of intelligence and expectations and overly high demands, it should be reasonable to diagnose ADHD/DAMP.

There is a need for a more well-considered policy for these issues in the future so that children who would benefit from certain types of intervention do not miss out on these because they lack a particular diagnosis. While it is true that one should treat the problems and not the diagnosis, sadly, experience clearly shows that a specific diagnosis—in the sense of ADHD, DAMP, or another named ESSENCE category—is often a prerequisite for satisfactory treatment. To simply list the problems without summarizing them under the umbrella of a diagnostic term rarely leads to optimal intervention measures in clinical practice.

In this context it is also important to stress that many children with mild IDD—or even intelligence within the low-normal range—encounter so many failures in today's society that they get all manner of mental problems, everything from acting out to depression and anxiety. Occasionally the question then arises whether ADHD/DAMP could be the root cause. A medical examination and a psychological evaluation can generally provide adequate information. Many parents seem to prefer an ADHD/DAMP diagnosis over one that states the child's intellectual disability as the primary problem. This may seem to be inconsequential, but one must still stress the importance of giving the most accurate diagnosis possible.

Intellectual problems (mild IDD and borderline intellectual functioning) are currently under diagnosed in the Western world (Fernell & Ek, 2010; Holmberg et al., 2005). For instance, there are from time to time 10-year-old children referred to child psychiatrists described with the preliminary diagnosis "bullying, depression." Examination including a neuropsychological test (among other things) then shows that the child's IQ is around 60 and that the "real" diagnosis is "mild IDD." After placement in an appropriate group with individually adjusted pedagogic needs, it doesn't take long before the depression is gone and the bullying has ceased.

TOURETTE SYNDROME AND OTHER TIC DISORDERS

In cases of Tourette syndrome there is a co-occurrence—according to the definition given in, for example, the DSM—of motor tics and one or more vocal tics (Robertson, 2012). In the majority of cases there are also sensory tics, and the individual may feel he or she has to act/react with a motor or vocal tic to the sensory phenomenon.

The different kinds of tics do not necessarily have to coincide, and the severity of the symptoms can vary greatly within the same individual, even from day to day. Periodically they can be very troublesome, but sometimes they can be mild (even "concealed") for months or sometimes years. The condition is, however, generally permanent in the sense that tics of different kinds rarely completely disappear for good, but can resurface during periods of both stress (including throat infections) and relaxation, or in other cases where one cannot discern any triggering factor. Tourette syndrome is usually caused by genes or the combination of genes and an environmental factor, and it can be triggered by some types of infections. In some such cases where an infection either triggers or exacerbates tic and obsessive-compulsive problems, the onset of severe symptoms can be very acute, emerging over a day or two or even from one hour to another. It is in these cases that the question of PANDAS most often arises (also now referred to as PANS [pediatric acute-onset neuropsychiatric syndrome]; see below).

The majority of individuals with Tourette syndrome also have problems with obsessive-compulsive syndromes of different kinds. The link with obsessive-compulsive symptoms is well documented and clinically significant. Many individuals with Tourette syndrome also meet the criteria for the diagnosis OCD according to the DSM. One form of compulsion in combination with lacking impulse control manifests in certain people with Tourette syndrome as what is referred to as coprolalia, an obsessive-compulsive uttering of bad words (e.g., curse words, long strings of profanities). Sometimes coprolalia and lack of impulse control manifest more extremely through anal and sex fixation. Some people with Tourette syndrome think obsessively about sex for large parts of the day and are sometimes unable to halt their impulses, neither verbally nor in action. Some recount—often wound up in an almost detached manner—bizarre sex stories. Others are drawn in an obsessive-compulsive and often not in a particularly excited manner to sex on TV, video, or the Internet. A very few people with Tourette syndrome cannot control impulses to expose themselves. In rare cases this kind of compulsion begins as early as the preschool years or early school years.

The perception of the rate of coprolalia and sexually charged obsessive-compulsive actions in cases of Tourette syndrome is a subject of great divide among researchers: some claim that they occur in the majority, others that they occur in only about 10% to 20%. Another variant verbal compulsion manifests as so-called palilalia, the obsessive-compulsive repetition of one's own sounds, words, and sentences. An obsessive-compulsive humming and whistling is also relatively common.

Problems with lack of attention and impulse control are also extremely common in tic disorders. Some studies indicate that around half of all people with Tourette syndrome meet the criteria for ADHD. In particular, lacking impulse control is very common in cases of Tourette syndrome. It is not uncommon for individuals meeting the criteria for Tourette syndrome also to meet the full criteria for both OCD and ADHD. In fact, it would be very unusual for somebody with Tourette syndrome not to also meet the criteria for either of the two additional diagnoses. It is very rare for the main impairing symptoms in clinical cases of Tourette syndrome not to be in the field of obsessive-compulsive or inattentive-hyperactive-impulsive behaviors. ADHD and OCD medications and cognitive-behavioral therapies effective for these disorders are the mainstay of treatments in tic disorders; neuroleptics effective for the tic symptoms are much more rarely used.

Sleep problems seem to occur at an increased rate in cases of Tourette syndrome; not least is it common for the person to have a warped or even reversed circadian rhythm.

Tourette syndrome occurs to such a pronounced degree that it causes personal suffering in about one in 100 children, and four to 10 times as often in boys as in girls. According to American, English, and Swedish studies, 1% of all schoolchildren have a combination of multiple motor tics and vocal tics (e.g., Kadesjö & Gillberg, 2000). Milder variants of Tourette syndrome are prevalent in a significantly larger group of children, adolescents, and adults. Experience from everyday life suggests that the rate could be even higher. Whether diagnosis should be given or not depends on whether the symptoms cause suffering or difficulty adjusting.

If someone has only motor tics or only vocal tics, regardless of how many, and has never had the other variant of tics, one does not refer to it as Tourette syndrome. This is sometimes a problem because someone with, for example, severe vocal tics, such as obsessive-compulsive loud barking noises, could be handicapped to an equally significant extent as someone with winking tics, shrugs, and relatively mild throat-clears who thus meets the criteria for the Tourette diagnosis. Still, it does not appear as though the problem would be of the same severity if one were to talk about "simple motor tics" or "simple vocal tics," which are the diagnostic terms used when the different variants of tics occur separately. Such simple tics occur in many people in the population. One in 10 children from the age of 5 to 12 have had tics, to a more or less bothersome extent.

There are additional problems with distinguishing between simple tics and Tourette syndrome. Research suggests that tics and Tourette syndrome are usually manifestations of the same genetic abnormality. Furthermore, there is not anything to suggest that the combination of motor and vocal tics constitutes anything specific other than that the person who has them has a central nervous system that predisposes him or her to different forms of tics and likely also to different types of obsessive-compulsive disorder.

Limited research suggests that Tourette syndrome could be associated with autism spectrum disorders in some cases. There are several reports on the co-occurrence of Asperger syndrome and Tourette syndrome/tics (Ehlers & Gillberg, 1993; Robertson, 2012).

Tics can only be partially suppressed through willpower. Some people manage to keep their tics in check in social situations and "explode" with tics when they are alone, for instance when going to the bathroom or before going to bed. The tics decrease in rate and magnitude, but do not always disappear entirely, while sleeping.

Motor tics and to some extent vocal tics are also suppressed by certain medicines, for example neuroleptics. These can be useful in very severe cases of disabling tics, or for temporary use such as in conjunction with a job interview and in similar situations. The side effects of neuroleptics are otherwise potentially so serious that one should not resort to them in "average" Tourette syndrome cases.

The majority of people with disabling forms of Tourette syndrome and severe "simple tics," however, have such severe obsessive-compulsive actions and sometimes also obsessive-compulsive thoughts that it may be reasonable to try treatment with medication, for example from the group of serotonin reuptake inhibitors (SRI drugs or clomipramine). It is important to point out that in this context, as in other cases, it is not the diagnosis itself that is to be treated, but the person's symptoms that might need to be alleviated through the help of medication or otherwise. The most disabling problems for children and adolescents with Tourette syndrome are often those that are linked with ADHD and obsessive-compulsiveness. ADHD in Tourette syndrome often needs the same kind of overall intervention approach that is recommended for ADHD without tics. Tics are not generally negatively affected by ADHD treatments, stimulant or non-stimulant.

OCD

OCD has been mentioned as a common coexisting disorder/problem in tic disorders, including in Tourette syndrome, and tic disorders are still often flagged up as *the* typical "OCD comorbidity" and vice versa. However, in young children who present with obsessive-compulsive symptoms (OCS) before age 10 years, the presenting problem (even before the onset of the OCS) is very often separation anxiety disorder, followed by ADHD (de Mathis et al., 2013). It is well established that when tic disorders are impairing it is very often because of the coexistence with either OCD or ADHD or both. It is less well recognized that, in some cases of early-onset ADHD (without tics), OCS/OCD, with time, can become some of the most impairing problems. Some authors—and indeed some patients— consider the development of OCS to be a "reaction" to hyperactivity and impulsivity.

The strong relationship between adult drug use/abuse and ADHD has been well documented. One report suggested that heroin addicts, like other drug abusers, have a very high rate of "underlying" ADHD (equally high in males and females) but also that, when ADHD is present, OCS are very often present at the same time (Peles et al., 2012).

ASD (AUTISM, ASPERGER SYNDROME, AND AUTISTIC TRAITS)

Autism is often seen as the most severe variant of a group of disorders hall-marked by major impairments in social communication and a rigid, stereo-typical behavioral phenotype (Gillberg, 1991; Coleman & Gillberg, 2012). Asperger syndrome is usually considered to be a mild variant of autism or otherwise as autism in individuals of average or above-average intelligence (Gillberg, 1991; Gillberg & Gillberg, 1989a). Autistic traits are those symp-toms within the so-called autism spectrum that are strongly reminiscent of those seen in cases of autism but do not occur to such a pronounced degree or in such typical constellations that the diagnoses of autism and Asperger syndrome are considered. Autism and Asperger syndrome (and other autistic-like conditions, including so-called pervasive developmen-tal disorder not otherwise specified) are increasingly subsumed under the common label of ASD. Autistic traits may also be included under an autism spectrum umbrella term, perhaps particularly when reference is made to "autism spectrum conditions." Clinicians and researchers nowadays often do not distinguish between the various clinical phenotypes within this spectrum and refer more generally to "ASD." The reasons for this include the lack of clear distinguishing background features, symptoms, outcomes, or intervention recommendations for the various purported subtypes of ASD. All the different types of ASD (including autistic traits) show a very high degree of heritability, but it is likely that epigenetic factors play some role in many cases (Delorme et al., 2013).

The full presentation of symptoms associated with the DSM/ICD category of ASD or the "older" category of childhood autism is usually not present in ADHD. The other clinical variants mentioned above, on the other hand, are very common, and one should expect even quite marked autistic traits in about one in four of all children with clinically impairing ADHD.

The clinical presentation of Asperger syndrome (such as the phenotype originally described by Hans Asperger in 1944) usually is one in which the following symptoms manifest coincidentally in one and the same child (Gillberg & Gillberg, 1989a) (see also Table 3.4.):

1. Impairment in social behavior dominated by extreme egocentricity with difficulties or lack of interest in playing with peers, lacking empathy and socially and emotionally inappropriate behavior.

2. Engrossing special interests with a strong tendency toward repetition and building rather than content and meaning.

3. Routines or ritual compulsion that control one's own life or the lives of others.

4. Idiosyncrasies in spoken language, which may have been delayed but is later generally perfect on the surface and characterized by monotonous voice or otherwise abnormal prosody. There is an excessive degree of formality, a lack of pragmatism, and a lack of comprehension of the fact that spoken language can mean different things depending on the context.

5. Idiosyncrasies in the nonverbal communication, such as
    staring gaze, limited facial expression and strange gestures,
    peculiar physical posture, and inability to gauge appropriate
    distance upon interacting with other people.

6. Abnormal or immature motor control characterized by
    clumsiness, often with a degree of stiffness, not least in social
    situations.

In order for an ASD diagnosis of the Asperger syndrome type to be
considered, these symptoms must cause significant difficulties in everyday
life or adjusting. Some people who have poor empathy, a lack of interest in
social interactions, and special interests are strongly reminiscent of those
diagnosed with Asperger syndrome, but they do not have enough problems to be disabled or to create difficulties for the people around them. It
is likely that they are in the same spectrum as those diagnosed with the
syndrome, but in practice it is not meaningful to give a diagnosis because
there is not any actual need of help. Such autistic traits are very common
in the general population, and up to 5% of school-age children have quite
marked features of autism without being socially or academically impaired
by them in any major way.

The diagnosis of Asperger syndrome is usually not given if all of the criteria for autism are met. An actual autism (or "autistic disorder"/"autistic syndrome") diagnosis points to a more severe disorder, which can require greater
supporting measures, and children and family are generally better served by
the autism diagnosis in such a case. However, not rarely does it occur that a
child who early in life met all the criteria for autism—and was therefore given
that diagnosis—later, for example upon reaching school years, fits the criteria for Asperger syndrome almost perfectly. It can then be reasonable to use
this term instead, among other things to highlight the progress that has been
made and the alleviation of the set of symptoms seen before. Alternatively, a
diagnosis of ASD is "applied" throughout the child's developmental period,
and the severity of the condition can be separately addressed; in such cases
the child's problems could be described as severe ASD in early childhood but
as moderate or mild ASD in adolescence (or vice versa).

As has been mentioned earlier, about three to four out of every 1,000 children who are born have the difficulties that the diagnosis of Asperger syndrome refers to. Boys are affected around four times as often as girls. The condition occurs in all levels of society and is *relatively* unaffected by environment. This does not mean that social factors are irrelevant, but that such factors mean little in shaping how the basic symptoms manifest. The majority with Asperger syndrome, however, are not noticed as being clearly abnormal before reaching their school years, and the diagnosis is often not given until the age of 8 to 12 or even later. The autism diagnosis, on the other hand, is generally given before the age of 5.

The delineation between severe ADHD/DAMP and autistic traits can sometimes be problematic. Many children with severe DAMP (i.e., those with ADHD, severe DCD, and speech and language problems) have mild to moderately severe autistic traits or autistic-like conditions, and the diagnoses can very well occur coincidentally. In some cases the autistic traits are so prominent that all the criteria for Asperger syndrome are met. In those cases it can be difficult to determine which of the diagnoses— ADHD, DAMP, or Asperger syndrome—should be given precedence as the main diagnosis (i.e., the diagnosis that best indicates which symptoms and problems are most important). In other cases it is doubtful whether one should really give both diagnoses.

The fact is that the majority of children with Asperger syndrome have *symptoms* (including some attention and hyperactivity problems, and motor control difficulties) that could lead to the need for a workup with a view to including/excluding a diagnosis of mild or moderate DAMP. Still, the child and family would usually not have any use for the additional diagnosis of DAMP in many of these cases. If, however, the difficulties in concentration and the problems with motor control and perception are so pronounced that they demand separate measures, an "extra" ADHD, DCD, or DAMP diagnosis could be called for. The most important thing is for everyone involved—parents, teachers, and maybe the child himself or herself—to have adequate knowledge of Asperger syndrome *and* ADHD/ DAMP (and of the other ESSENCE categories) so they understand that it is often not a question of it being either/or, but rather a little or a lot of both (or more than two "disorders") in most children affected by one ESSENCE condition.

Asperger syndrome and autistic traits are not usually fundamentally affected by any medical or psychological therapies. Nevertheless, both intervention methods can occasionally be called for to improve the quality of life, particularly when problems relating to sleep or obsessive and violent behaviors dominate the clinical presentation. Special education and applied behavioral analytic methods where one stresses structure, concretization, predictability, enhanced communication, and monotony can be very valuable and should be considered in all cases.

PANDAS/PANS AND OTHER ACUTE ONSET SYMPTOMS

Acute onset of obsessive compulsive symptoms, anxiety, tics, ADHD symptoms, and autistic symptoms in any combination can be a dramatic experience for children and adolescents and their families. They have, from time to time, been associated with autoimmune processes and various kinds of coccal (including streptococcal) infections. PANDAS, more recently referred to as PANS, is still a controversial concept in many centers, but there is growing support for its validity, and the clinical empirical evidence clearly supports an acute-onset neuropsychiatric syndrome that can include most of the behavioral and cognitive problems subsumed under the ESSENCE umbrella (Dale & Vincent, 2010; Hoekstra et al., 2013) (Table 9.1).

At onset, symptoms may have followed an asymptomatic/untreated/unnoticed streptococcal infection by several months or longer. However, on subsequent infection recurrences, the worsening of the neuropsychiatric symptoms may be the first sign of an occult ("hidden") strep infection. Prompt treatment of the strep infection is often effective in reducing the OCD and other neuropsychiatric symptoms.

Strep throat infections can be diagnosed only by obtaining a throat culture that yields group A beta-hemolytic streptococcal bacteria. To have a reliable throat culture, the swab must reach the oropharynx, which

TABLE 9.1.
DIAGNOSTIC CRITERIA FOR PANDAS ACCORDING TO NIMH (2013)

1. Presence of clinically significant obsessions, compulsions, and/or tics*
2. Unusually abrupt (24–48 hours) onset of symptoms or a relapsing-remitting course of symptom severity
3. Prepubertal onset
4. Association with other neuropsychiatric symptoms (ADHD, anxiety, sensory overreactions, irritability, depression, regression, and increased urinary frequency)
5. Association with streptococcal infection**

* Other neuropsychiatric symptoms might well usher in the syndrome.
** Other coccal or infectious agents are sometimes involved.

typically is slightly uncomfortable and makes the child gag. A throat culture swab that touches only the back of the tongue will give a falsely negative result, as will one that is just touched to the sides of the throat. Poorly done throat cultures are a very common cause of false-negative results. Rapid strep tests can also give false-negative results, as they miss about 15% of cases. If the rapid strep test is negative, an overnight culture should be done to make sure that there aren't strep bacteria present.

Antistreptococcal titers can also be used to diagnose a strep throat but require that two separate blood tests are done several weeks apart and are timed just right to show a "rising titer." Strep infections trigger the production of antistreptococcal antibodies, which are measured by the titers. When the child is initially infected with the strep bacteria, the titers will be low, but they should increase over the next 4 to 6 weeks as more antistreptococcal antibodies are produced. If the child's blood is tested too late, the titers may already be elevated, but it won't be possible to know if these "high titers" are related to the current difficulties or if they're left over from a previous strep infection, since titers can remain elevated for several months or longer. Thus, a single "high antistreptococcal antibody titer" isn't sufficient to prove that a strep infection was the trigger for the child's symptoms.

PANS has more recently been postulated as an umbrella term intended to be broader than PANDAS, including not only disorders potentially associated with a preceding infection but also acute-onset neuropsychiatric disorders without an apparent environmental precipitant or immune dysfunction. Because cases of PANS are defined clinically, the syndrome is expected to include a number of related disorders that have different etiologies but share a common clinical presentation—"the foudroyant (lightning-like) onset or recurrence of OCD which is accompanied by two or more co-occurring neuropsychiatric symptoms" (Swedo et al., 2012).

It is important to recognize that other, seemingly acute onset disorders, including X-linked adenoleukodystrophy and early symptomatic Huntington's chorea can present with the combination of ADHD, OCD and anxiety disorders.

DEPRESSION

Depression is common among people with ADHD/DAMP (Gillberg & Gillberg, 1983, 1989b). It is, however, important to note that depression in a person who does not have ADHD/DAMP can be misinterpreted as ADHD/DAMP, even if this happens much more rarely than ADHD/DAMP going unnoticed in cases of depression (Barkley & Brown, 2008).

Depression often brings about difficulties in concentration, memory problems, inattention, and awkward motor control, symptoms that are all common in ADHD/DAMP. The difference is that in ADHD/DAMP, the symptoms have existed for years and thus have not appeared just recently. In addition, in cases of ADHD/DAMP, despite the awkward motor control, there are usually not motor control/perception symptoms of the same kind as among people with DAMP.

Depression in young children and adolescents often primarily manifests as a sudden or relatively sudden change in the person's behavior (Luby 2010). It can be a matter of decreased as well as increased activity; the change itself is a more important signal symptom than in which direction the behavior changes. Generally one notices relatively soon that there are other symptoms as well. Fatigue, increased or diminished appetite, more or less sleep, feeling frozen, and constipation are all common problems associated with depression that can indicate that the hypothalamic nuclei in the brain—with a central role in production and regulation of a variety of hormones, including those strongly related to stress—are not working optimally (Luby et al., 2003).

Depression in children, with or without ADHD/DAMP, is much more common than was once believed, and it is a condition for which the rate has probably increased over the past 40 years. However, the knowledge of where one should draw the line for a depression diagnosis is much too limited for any exact percentages to be mentioned when discussing the prevalence of depression among young people.

The underlying cause of depression is often a complex interaction between a variety of different factors—social, psychological, genetic, and epigenetic (Luby et al., 2003). In a select few cases the causes can surely be more one-sided and clearly defined, but many times it is a matter of a number of different negative factors working together. The link between neurological and neuropsychiatric disorders and secondary depressed mood has been noted during the past few years. In many cases it is reasonable to see the depression as a state of helplessness, of not being able to do anything about one's own situation. Not just ADHD/DAMP but other disorders and life situations can lead to a state of helplessness, despondency, and hopelessness that could very well lead to a depression.

Depression in children and adolescents can be treated with psychological and medical methods, often in tandem. Negative social and psychological factors, for example bullying and other kinds of abuse, must be dealt with primarily. Adding antidepressants can occasionally be helpful.

BIPOLAR DISORDER

Bipolar disorder was long considered to occur only from puberty onward. However, in recent years it has become apparent that manic-depressive illness can manifest as early as the first years of life, usually in families with diagnosed manic-depressive disorder. Children with very severe mood swings, a high irritability level, easily triggered aggression, and extreme hyperactivity/impulsiveness could have a bipolar disorder. Such children may or may not have been thought of or even diagnosed as having ADHD before a diagnosis of bipolar disorder is considered. The probability increases if a close relative has been diagnosed with manic-depressive or bipolar disorder. Noticeable periodicity is prevalent in some cases but is not as prominent as during adulthood.

There is an ongoing debate as to how common it is for ADHD to "antedate" bipolar disorder and to what extent the two overlap or can sometimes be seen as different aspects of the same underlying disorder. The evidence so far does not suggest shared heritability (Landaas et al., 2011), and the results from large-scale systematic studies are compatible with ADHD and bipolar disorder being separately heritable.

OTHER SEVERE MENTAL OR NEUROLOGICAL PROBLEMS

Difficulties in concentration, inability to stay put, poor attention, and difficulties in memory can be symptoms of just about any mental illness or disorder. Occasionally they can be manifestations of a severe and possibly progressive neurological disorder. This is one of the most important reasons why children with ADHD/DAMP and other ESSENCE must always be examined and diagnosed by doctors.

Cerebral palsy is a diagnosis for a group of motor disorders that entail certain types of difficulties in motor control as a result of an injury or disorder in the brain that has arisen very early in life (usually during fetal development) and which is, in principle, an isolated incident. Depending on the examination of the difficulties in motor control, different syndromes of cerebral palsy are described. About half of the children with cerebral palsy also suffer from IDD. In many, also among those who do not have IDD, there are significant difficulties in concentration, stamina, activity, and impulse control and also perception disorders. This means that many children with cerebral palsy also have symptoms of ADHD/

DAMP (Surén et al., 2012), even if, in accordance with the diagnostic criteria, this may not lead to ADHD/DAMP diagnoses being given.

The line between cerebral palsy and DCD can sometimes be very thin. Within the ADHD group, and above all within the group with severe DAMP, approximately 20% have very pronounced difficulties in motor control. The majority of these have difficulties due to an abnormal motor control that differs from the problems with motor control seen in the majority of children with DAMP. To an extent, the larger group with DCD (in DAMP; i.e., in ADHD + DCD) can at least partly be described in terms of immaturity and difficulties in coordination, whereas the 20% group resembles a mild version of cerebral palsy.

Upon closer analysis of the deviations in motor control found in cases of severe DAMP, one occasionally (rarely) finds that they are strongly reminiscent of the deviations found in one of the cerebral palsy syndromes. It can then be reasonable to refer to it as "minimal cerebral palsy." The most common variants are made up of *minimal ataxia* (balance and coordination disorder), *minimal diplegia* (coordination disorder combined with high muscle tone and elevated reflexes mainly in the legs), and *minimal hemiplegia* (coordination disorder combined with high muscle tone and elevated reflexes in the left or right extremities).

Certain muscle diseases (muscular dystrophy) and disorders in the peripheral nerves (polyneuropathy) can sometimes, particularly at an early stage, manifest as a problem with motor control similar to those seen among people with ADHD/DAMP. They often also have presenting cognitive and/or behavioral problems, including inattention, impulsivity, hyperactivity, and autistic features. For this reason—so that such diseases will not be incorrectly diagnosed as ADHD/DAMP "only"—it is important that every child with symptoms of ADHD/DAMP be examined by a medical doctor (with some training in neurology).

Children with cerebral palsy fairly often have mental problems of different kinds, including, even on presentation, difficulties strongly reminiscent of those seen in cases of ADHD/DAMP. According to the diagnostic criteria for ADHD/DAMP such a diagnosis should not be given in those cases. In everyday life, however, it is not entirely uncommon for exceptions to be made to this protocol. Sometimes the exception is motivated by a need to treat, for example, difficulties in concentration and hyperactivity with the help of medication.

CONCLUDING REMARKS

ADHD can be confused with a variety of other conditions, and many conditions can appear coincidentally with ADHD. The most common problem types one must be well aware of in order to be able to make a correct distinction vis-à-vis ADHD (or more commonly, a comorbid diagnosis *with* ADHD) are ODD and DCD (although both can be seen as "part and parcel" of particular subgroups of ADHD), difficulties in reading and writing, IDD, tics and Tourette syndrome, Asperger syndrome and autistic traits in general, depression, bipolar disorder, and, in a small number of cases, more severe forms of disability in terms of motor control, including cerebral palsy, muscular dystrophy, and polyneuropathy.

REFERENCES

Barkley, R.A., & Brown, T.E. (2008). Unrecognized attention-deficit/hyperactivity disorder in adults presenting with other psychiatric disorders. *CNS Spectrums, 13,* 977–984.

Coleman, M., & Gillberg, C. (2012). *The autisms* (4th ed.). New York: Oxford University Press.

Dale, R.C., & Vincent, A. (Eds.). (2010). *Inflammatory and autoimmune disorders of the nervous system in children.* London: Mac Keith Press.

Delorme, R., Ey, E., Toro, R., Leboyer, M., Gillberg, C., & Bourgeron, T. (2013) Progress toward treatments for synaptic defects in autism. *Nature Medicine, 19,* 685–694.

de Mathis, M.A., Diniz, J.B., Hounie, A.G., Shavitt, R.G., Fossaluza, V., Ferrão, Y., et al. (2013). Trajectory in obsessive-compulsive disorder comorbidities. *European Neuropsychopharmacology, 23, 594–601.*

Ehlers, S., & Gillberg, C. (1993). The epidemiology of Asperger syndrome. A total population study. *Journal of Child Psychology and Psychiatry, 34,* 1327–1350.

Fernell, E., & Ek, U. (2010). Borderline intellectual functioning in children and adolescents—insufficiently recognized difficulties. *Acta Paediatrica, 99,* 748–753.

Gillberg, C. (1991). Clinical and neurobiological aspects of Asperger syndrome in six family studies. In U. Frith (Ed.), *Autism and Asperger syndrome* (pp. 122–146). New York: Cambridge University Press.

Gillberg, C. (2010). The ESSENCE in child psychiatry: early symptomatic syndromes eliciting neurodevelopmental clinical examinations. *Research in Developmental Disabilities, 31,* 1543–1551.

Gillberg, I.C., & Gillberg, C. (1983). Three-year follow-up at age 10 of children with minor neurodevelopmental disorders. I: Behavioural problems. *Developmental Medicine and Child Neurology, 25,* 438–449.

Gillberg, I.C., & Gillberg, C. (1989a). Asperger syndrome—some epidemiological considerations: a research note. *Journal of Child Psychology and Psychiatry, 30,* 631–638.

Gillberg, I.C., & Gillberg, C. (1989b). Children with preschool minor neurodevelopmental disorders. IV: Behaviour and school achievement at age 13. *Developmental Medicine and Child Neurology, 31,* 3–13.

Hoekstra, P.J., Dietrich, A., Edwards, M.J., Elamin, I., & Martino, D. (2013). Environmental factors in Tourette syndrome. *Neuroscience and Biobehavioral Reviews, 37*(6), 1040–1049.

Holmberg, K., Bråkenhielm, G., Norrman, B., & Fernell, E. (2005). [Children with mild mental retardation in the special schools. "Top of the iceberg"?]. *Läkartidningen, 102,* 382–385.

Kadesjö, B., & Gillberg, C. (2000). Tourette's disorder: epidemiology and comorbidity in primary school children. *Journal of the American Academy of Child and Adolescent Psychiatry, 39,* 548–555.

Landaas, E.T., Johansson, S., Halmøy, A., Oedegaard, K.J., Fasmer, O.B., Haavik, J., et al. (2011). Bipolar disorder risk alleles in adult ADHD patients. *Genes, Brain, and Behavior, 10,* 418–423.

Luby, J.L. (2010). Preschool depression: the importance of identification of depression early in development. *Current Directions in Psychological Science, 10,* 91–95.

Luby, J.L., Heffelfinger, A., Mrakotsky, C., Brown, K., Hessler, M., & Spitznagel, E. (2003). Alterations in stress cortisol reactivity in depressed preschoolers relative to psychiatric and no-disorder comparison groups. *Archives of General Psychiatry, 60,* 1248–1255.

Neville, B. (2013). Role of ESSENCE for preschool children with neurodevelopmental disorders. *Brain & Development, 35*(2), 128–132.

Peles, E., Schreiber, S., Sutzman, A., & Adelson, M. (2012). Attention deficit hyperactivity disorder and obsessive-compulsive disorder in methadone maintenance treatment. *Psychopathology, 45,* 325–337.

Robertson, M.M. (2012) The Gilles de la Tourette syndrome: the current status. *Archives of Disease in Childhood, 97,* 166–175.

Surén, P., Bakken, I.J., Aase, H., Chin, R., Gunnes, N., Lie, K.K., et al. (2012). Autism spectrum disorder, ADHD, epilepsy, and cerebral palsy in Norwegian children. *Pediatrics, 130,* e152–e158.

Swedo, S.E, Leckman, J.F., & Rose, N.R. (2012). From research subgroup to clinical syndrome: modifying the PANDAS criteria to describe PANS (pediatric acute-onset neuropsychiatric syndrome). *Pediatrics & Therapeutics, 2,* 113.

Diagnosis of ADHD, DAMP, or Disorders in ESSENCE Group

ADHD, DAMP, and other ESSENCE are, much like cerebral palsy, neuromuscular disorders, and epilepsy, *medical diagnoses.* They cannot be "handed out" without the participation of a medically trained specialist doctor (Gillberg, 2010).

To form an adequate basis for establishing a diagnosis of ADHD, DAMP, or another one of the disorders in the ESSENCE group, an examination, by a doctor *and* a psychologist, both with intimate knowledge and experience of normal child and adolescent development, is required. The examination must—during the childhood and adolescent years—entail interviews between a doctor and whoever knows the child's development and behavior best—generally the mother, sometimes the father or another caretaker—*and* a medical examination of the child, including a neuro-psychiatric evaluation *and* a neuropsychological examination of the child. These examinations, complemented by questionnaires designed to get an idea of the child's behavior at home and at preschool/school, are enough to decide whether ADHD/DAMP diagnosis should be considered or not. In many cases, complementary examinations of different kinds, particularly by education specialists, are needed.

INTERVIEWING THE PARENT

The physician's interview with the mother or other close caretaker (such as the father) is aimed at generating:

1. A description of the child's current behavior, adjustment, and mental functions in general
2. An overall picture of how the child has developed up until the time of the examination
3. Information on diseases and traumatic experiences of different kinds
4. The current situation regarding family, preschool/school, peers, and wider social network

If the child is around the age of 3 to 10 years old at the time of the consultation, it is helpful to get specific information regarding his or her current ability to concentrate, gross and fine motor skills, as well as the developmental rate within these areas (Rasmussen et al., 1983) (Tables 10.1 and 10.2).

EXAMINATION OF THE CHILD

The examination of the child should include a general physical examination (including, always, weight, height, head circumference, speech, hearing, and visual screens, skin inspection, and assessment for the presence of minor physical anomalies) plus a neurological/motor skills evaluation (Gillberg et al., 1982) (Table 10.3).

The medical examination should also form the basis of preliminary stances regarding the prevalence of coincidental/alternative diagnoses such as depression, DCD, IDD, ASD, tics, and Tourette syndrome. When interviewing the mother and child as well as during the direct examination of the child, the doctor must keep these problem areas in mind and must have adequate knowledge to be able to decide whether additional

TABLE 10.1.
QUESTIONS TO PARENT AT MEDICAL EXAMINATION OF CHILDREN AGED
ABOUT 3 TO 10 YEARS

Ask the following six questions and get the parent to compare the child with

other children:

1. What was your child's language development like?

2. What was your child's general development of motor skills like?

3. What are your child's gross motor skills like (e.g., while walking, running,

   climbing, jumping on one leg, etc.)?

4. What are your child's fine motor skills like (e.g., while drawing, cutting,

   buttoning, eating, etc.)?

5. Did your child move about in an unusual way (e.g., by "dragging" his/her

   bottom/"shuffling" across the floor) before learning to walk?

6. Does your child have problems concentrating/"listening" or is he/she

   particularly hyperactive or impulsive?

If the response to any of these six questions leads to concern that development

or behavior might be problematic, then it is usually relevant to make a fuller

assessment. Other relevant questions to ask can be checked by using the

ESSENCE-Q (Gillberg, 2013), a one-page questionnaire that can be completed

by parents of children of any age (Table 10.2). This is often best delivered while

the parent is in the waiting room and can then be gone over when the doctor

interviews the parent soon after.

examinations are necessary to determine whether such "additional problems" exist or not.

NEUROPSYCHOLOGICAL EVALUATION

The neuropsychological evaluation should include an examination with
one of the Wechsler scales (WPPSI, WISC, or WAIS, depending on
the patient's age) or another appropriate scale, providing information
about general intelligence level and whether or not the profile is the one
believed to be "characteristic" for underlying working memory/speed

TABLE 10.2.
THE ESSENCE-Q (GILLBERG, 2013) FOR USE BY PARENTS OF CHILDREN
OF ANY AGE

ESSENCE-Q			
Name of child:			
Age:	Gender:	Completed by:	Date:

Please take a few minutes to read and check the following items. Have you
(or anybody else, who?_____) been concerned for more than a few
months regarding child's development?

Y= Yes   M/AL = Maybe/A little   N=No

	Y	M/AL	N
1. General development	☐	☐	☐
2. Motor development/milestones	☐	☐	☐
3. Sensory reactions (e.g., touch, sound, light, smell, taste, heat, cold, pain)	☐	☐	☐
4. Communication/language/babble	☐	☐	☐
5. Activity (overactivity/passivity) or impulsivity	☐	☐	☐
6. Attention/concentration/"listening"	☐	☐	☐
7. Social interaction/interest in other children	☐	☐	☐
8. Behavior (e.g., repetitive, routine insistence)	☐	☐	☐
9. Mood (depressed, elated/manic, extreme irritability, crying spells)	☐	☐	☐
10. Sleep	☐	☐	☐
11. Feeding	☐	☐	☐
12. "Funny spells"/absences	☐	☐	☐

If Y or M/AL to any of the above, please elaborate briefly here:
The ESSENCE-Q will help draw attention to virtually all the potentially
problematic areas in children who raise suspicion of suffering from ADHD,
DAMP, or any of the other named syndromes subsumed under the ESSENCE
acronym. If a parent responds with an affirmative Yes for any of the 12 listed
items, or with a Maybe/A little for two or more of them, then this would definitely
mean that the areas listed as of any concern would have to be gone through in
much more detail during the interview.

(continued)

TABLE 10.2.
(CONTINUED)

The family history must be reviewed in detail. It is common for ADHD/DAMP and other ESSENCE to be familial, and a thorough anamnesis (previous history) is crucial in order to draw a reasonable conclusion as to the cause of the current problems. Oftentimes one must discuss this issue again upon a return visit when the parent will have had time to think about the child's problems as well as their own, and the behavior, difficulties, and possible symptoms of the closest relatives, in the new light that the awareness of the child's diagnosis brings.
In conjunction with the interview with the physician, one should discuss the situation during the pregnancy and delivery using medical records as a reference point. Injuries during fetal development and the first year of life are sometimes the cause, or a contributing factor, in cases of ADHD/DAMP (or any other ESSENCE for that matter). For requisition of medical records from the maternity clinic and delivery ward, and any possible records from when the child has been in care at the newborn ward or child clinic, the parent's written permission is required.

processing problems often seen in ADHD/DAMP or not (Nydén et al., 2000) (Table 10.4). In over 90% of all cases it is adequate, with this limited neuropsychological examination, along with what was gleaned from the interview between the physician and the mother and from the examination of the child, to definitely determine whether or not the diagnosis ADHD/DAMP applies—and also to decide which other diagnoses should be considered, not least IDD and/or ASD.

In some severe or complex cases a more extensive neuropsychological examination is needed, for example portions of the (or the whole) NEPSY (Korkman et al., 2007), the QB test (Ulberstad, 2012), and/or other attention, empathy, speech/language tests. Even in some mild cases with complex psychosocial or medical problems, the neuropsychological examination may sometimes have to be expanded. Specific tests of reading and writing must be used to be able to diagnose coexisting dyslexia. At all schools there must be a specifically trained special pedagogue/teacher who can perform such tests.

TABLE 10.3.
CHILD MOTOR FUNCTIONING EXAMINATION CHART WITH INDICATION OF
CUTOFF FOR ABNORMALITY FOR YOUNG SCHOOL-AGE CHILDREN

1. Jump 20 times on one leg, one side at a time. Abnormality exists if this takes equal to or more than 12 seconds to complete on either side or if the child must use the other foot for "support" 2 or more times.
2. Stand on one leg for 20 seconds, one side at a time. Result is abnormal if the child manages 10 seconds or less on either side.
3. Walk on the lateral sides of the feet for 10 seconds (Fogs' test) with hands hanging down and swinging. Demonstrate! Result is abnormal in terms of accompanying movements if the elbow is bent 60 degrees or more on either side or in case of marked shoulder abduction or movements of lip and tongue or in case of noticeable asymmetry.
4. Rapidly alternating pro-supination (turning upside-down) of each hand separately for 10 seconds. Demonstrate by bending the child's elbow at 90 degrees, holding it out a bit away from the child's body, and, by "taking his/her hand" and twisting back and forth, show the motion itself. Abnormality is present if the child manages 10 pro-supinations or less on either side or if the motion occurs without any "flow" to it and the elbow moves sideways 15 centimetres (6 inches) or more.
5. Cut out a circle with a diameter of 1 decimetre (4 inches) from a semi-stiff paper. The result is considered abnormal if one fifth or more of the circle's surface has been cut out of the circle or if a surface of paper equivalent to one fifth or more of the circle's surface is included outside the circle or if it takes the child 2 minutes or more to cut out the circle.
6. The labyrinth part of the WISC-R test according to the manual's instructions. This is very easy to complete and only takes a few minutes. If the child can complete all the labyrinths (that are drawn on the same single sheet of paper) without errors, he/she gets 21 points. Result is abnormal if the score is 8 or less. Other labyrinth tests can be used.

TABLE 10.4.
TYPICAL WISC PROFILES IN CHILDREN WITH WORKING MEMORY AND
PROCESSING SPEED PROBLEMS, PARTICULARLY THOSE WHO MEET
CRITERIA FOR ADHD/DAMP, ASPERGER SYNDROME, OR AUTISTIC
DISORDER

Symptom/diagnosis "Typical" WISC profile (present only in about 50% of cases meeting symptom criteria for ADHD, 70% in Asperger syndrome, and 80% in autism)
Severe ADHD/DAMP
Very uneven profile
Low result on two or more of:
Coding/Digit Symbol
Digit Span
Arithmetic
Information
Mild ADHD/DAMP
Uneven profile
Low result on one or more of:
Coding/Digit Symbol
Digit Span
Arithmetic
Information
Asperger syndrome
High result on the overall verbal scale
Comprehension low in early-mid childhood
Comprehension often much better later
Low result on two or more of:
Coding/Digit Symbol
Arithmetic
Object Assembly
Picture Arrangement (more typical of older WISC-versions, see under Autism)
Autism
High result on:
Block Design
Low result on both:
Picture Arrangement (older, e.g. WISC-R, not necessarily low on WISC-III or IV where results rely more on visual perception than social context)
Comprehension

Depending on diagnosis and on what additional information has emerged during these examinations it can, of course, be necessary to perform more tests.

RATING OF THE CHILD'S BEHAVIOR BASED ON QUESTIONNAIRES

Some type of rating of the child's behavior through a questionnaire should be made in conjunction with diagnosis and at the time of follow-up. The different variants of the Conners behavior rating scales that work well for children in the preschool and primary school ages are especially useful. The brief Conners questionnaire (Conners, 1969), comprising 10 tasks, is especially easy to use and takes only about a minute or two to fill out (Table 10.5). This scale gives a good idea of the child's current level of activity, ability to concentrate, and impulse control. It can be administered to both the parent and (preferably through the parent) the teacher. The score range is 0 to 30 abnormality points, and 10 or more on both the parent and teacher rating are considered a sign of abnormality within the "attention area."

LABORATORY INVESTIGATIONS

For the majority of children with ADHD/DAMP the examinations described thus far are enough to form the basis for determining whether ADHD/DAMP is present or not.

In many cases of ADHD/DAMP it is necessary to add an EEG test. Subclinical epilepsy (i.e., changes on the EEG that correspond with those seen in cases of epilepsy but without clear signs of there existing any seizure episodes) and rare forms of epilepsy, such as certain types of absences, including so-called petit mal, can cause attention disorders that are difficult to diagnose. Symptoms of ADHD/DAMP can be the only thing alerting the people involved to an underlying epilepsy disorder. Treatment with antiepileptic medication can in some of these (rare) cases lead to the ADHD/DAMP problems disappearing.

Computerized reaction time meters can be valuable tools in the diagnostics and follow-up of children and adolescents with ADHD/DAMP and other ESSENCE. Various types of "continuous performance tests" exist for use on the computer; these include the Test of Visual Attention/ TOVA (Wada et al., 2000) and the QB test, both of which are available for use with both children and adults. The visual reaction time (i.e., the time it takes from the point when a visual stimulus is presented on a monitor to the point when the person presses a button) is often delayed in cases of ADHD/DAMP. When there are strong aspects of hyperactivity and impulsiveness the reaction time is sometimes normal or fast but the number of missed and incorrect button presses is high. When using different types of treatment—including those that involve medication—one can see how these variables can be affected positively. The child's confidence often increases when this can be demonstrated in as clear a manner as when using the reaction time meter.

Brain stem audiometry, magnetic resonance imaging (MRI), or a computed tomography scan (CT scan) of the brain, measuring of cerebral blood flow, blood and urine samples (including tests of thyroid function when ADHD is combined with a high or low heart rate or other signs of high or low metabolism) of different kinds can all be considered in special cases but are not normally necessary. Specific chromosome and gene tests (including for sex chromosome aneuploidies, 22q11del-syndrome and fragile X syndrome) will be needed if other indications (mental or physical) indicate the presence of a specific underlying genetic condition. Microarray analysis of the genome will probably be offered in quite a number of ESSENCE cases in clinics in the near future. In the section on brain damage in Chapter 10 there are additional opinions about which examinations could be considered in cases of DAMP.

A number of other examinations should be considered in special cases (Table 10.5). A physiotherapist and a child neurologist/child habilitation doctor may need to be brought in to assess the person's motor skills. Child (neuro) psychiatrists may need to be consulted for an evaluation

TABLE 10.5.
CONNERS BRIEF QUESTIONNAIRE REGARDING THE CHILD'S BEHAVIOR

Statement does not apply at all	Applies to a certain extent	Applies fairly well	Applies very well
1. Restless or hyperactive			
2. Is easily excited			
3. Disturbs other children			
4. Fails to finish activities that he/she has started—can only focus for a short amount of time			
5. Constantly moves about in an anxious/tumultuous manner			
6. Inattentive, easy to distract			
7. Needs must immediately be fulfilled—is easily made disappointed			
8. Quickly and often resorts to tears			
9. Rapid and violent mood swings			
10. Tantrums, explosive and unpredictable behavior			

of additional problems of different kinds. Such an evaluation can, however, sometimes wait until the family and school have had a semester or so to adjust to the new awareness of ADHD/DAMP. A speech therapist could be needed in cases of especially severe speech and language disorders.

WHO CAN PROVIDE THE DIAGNOSIS?

It is still not possible to point out any one group of specialists and say "people in that field can make the diagnosis." School doctors *should* have the competence, as should child psychiatrists, "community" or "behavioral" pediatricians, child neurologists, and habilitation doctors. Psychologists well trained in neuropsychology and pedagogues with a good understanding of dyslexia need to work in teams with these doctors within schools, community pediatrics, child psychiatry, and habilitation for the diagnostics to be meaningful and detailed enough for a reasonable plan of action to be suggested.

SCREENING—FOR WHOM?

Screening for ADHD/DAMP should—if it is to be done at all—be performed at the latest when the child is in the first or second grade of school. A screening for ADHD/DAMP does not, however, have to be so narrow as to pick up only on ADHD/DAMP problems but also dyslexia, borderline intelligence, IDD, ASD, and other serious ESSENCE problems.

Many, perhaps between a third and a half, of all with ADHD/DAMP have been spotted before starting school, usually because the family has sought help due to the child's abnormal behavior or late language development. It is not generally the case that the diagnosis is "correct" the first time around, but at least the difficulties have been noted.

For at least half, however, no diagnosis has been given by the time the child starts school. One would want a simple screening to pick up on the problems and lead to measures being taken before the child starts school. The problem is that if the screening is performed at preschool or at the child welfare center—and is not repeated at school—there is a great risk that information regarding the child's functional impairments and their consequences will never reach the school, or will reach it only in such a form that the meaning is lost. The best thing would be for a screening at the child welfare center to be done when the child is 5 to 6 years old and then another one in school around 2 years later. That way, one would minimize the risk of children with ADHD/DAMP staying undetected.

Unfortunately there is as of yet no foundation for any truly effective screening method for children below approximately 6 years of age. It is possible that screening for language delay around 2.5 years would pick up a very large proportion of *all* children with any type of problem within the ESSENCE group, but there is still a need for more research before this can be suggested as a general screening model for all Western countries. In a more long-term perspective one would prefer a more precise detection method that could be aimed at small preschool children. This, however, requires further research, and until such a method has been found, it is definitely time to introduce general screenings for children starting school. If resources are very limited it could be reasonable to concentrate the screenings to school health services. The most severe cases would then generally be detected—and ideally correctly diagnosed—before starting school, but many of the moderate cases would not be diagnosed until in conjunction with the school's screening.

One wonders whether screening causes children to be "singled out" and why it should be done "if the school does not have any resources to administer treatment anyway." However, this type of discussion usually misses the point: *children with ADHD/DAMP are already singled out,* as dumb, lazy, mean, and hopeless—not to mention the fact that many people with ADHD/DAMP have identified themselves as such. An accurate diagnosis, with hope for understanding, changes in attitude, and better adjustment of the pedagogy, can *never* make the situation worse. Anyone who wonders whether this is true can ask children and adolescents with ADHD/DAMP and their parents how they look at having been given the diagnosis. In the demand for "treatment measures before screening" (i.e., that one must be able to offer some kind of treatment after the diagnosis has been given), most people forget that a diagnosis is a form of treatment in itself. Having a name for the difficulties one is experiencing can never be worse than fumbling in the dark. The name also comes with information about causes, risks, and reasonable approaches. Even if—at worst—nothing else can be offered, that is still not a bad treatment effort!

CONCLUDING REMARKS

All children suspected of having ADHD/DAMP or another of the disorders in the ESSENCE group should be personally examined by a physician and a psychologist with training in neuropsychology. Taking a detailed medical/psychiatric history from at least one parent is necessary. A limited review of this kind is often sufficient to be able to confirm or reject the diagnosis. Further examinations, including with EEG, could be necessary. School health services and community/behavioral pediatrics should be able to handle the majority of young patients with mild and moderate

ADHD/DAMP, and screening should be performed during one of the first years of school. Child psychiatrists and habilitation doctors must be able to accept a relatively large portion of the severe ADHD/DAMP cases, and in addition develop and communicate new information about the whole ADHD/DAMP/ESSENCE field. Adults with previously undiagnosed ADHD/DAMP/ESSENCE will need to have access to good diagnostic and intervention services. This will lead to increasing demands—and a shift of focus—throughout general medicine and adult psychiatry. This is dealt with in more detail in a separate chapter.

REFERENCES

Conners, C.K. (1969). A teacher rating scale for use in drug studies with children. *American Journal of Psychiatry, 126,* 884–888.

Gillberg, C. (2010). The ESSENCE in child psychiatry: early symptomatic syndromes eliciting neurodevelopmental clinical examinations. *Research in Developmental Disabilities, 31,* 1543–1551.

Gillberg, C., Rasmussen, P., Carlström, G., Svenson, B., & Waldenström, E. (1982). Perceptual, motor and attentional deficits in six-year-old children. Epidemiological aspects. *Journal of Child Psychology and Psychiatry, 23,* 131–144.

Korkman, M., Kirk, U., & Kemp, S.L. (2007). *NEPSY II. Clinical and interpretative manual.* San Antonio, TX: Psychological Corporation.

Nydén, A., Hjelmquist, E., & Gillberg, C. (2000). Autism spectrum and attention-deficit disorders in girls. Some neuropsychological aspects. *European Child & Adolescent Psychiatry, 9,* 180–185.

Rasmussen, P., Gillberg, C., Waldenström, E., & Svenson, B. (1983). Perceptual, motor and attentional deficits in seven-year-old children: neurological and neurodevelopmental aspects. *Developmental Medicine and Child Neurology, 25,* 315–333.

Ulberstad, F. (2012). *Quantified behavioral test (QbTest) technical manual.* Stockholm, Sweden: Qbtech AB.

Wada, N., Yamashita, Y., Matsuishi, T., Ohtani, Y., & Kato, H. (2000). The Test of Variables of Attention (TOVA) is useful in the diagnosis of Japanese male children with attention deficit hyperactivity disorder. *Brain & Development, 22,* 378–382.

Causes, Risk Factors, and Laboratory Findings

ADHD is now considered a multifactorially determined condition with both genetic and environmental roots (Gillberg, 2010; Makris et al., 2009). MBD was originally viewed as a distinct "brain damage problem," but the consensus has now shifted to ADHD/DAMP—and most other ESSENCE—being regarded primarily as genetically driven sets of problems. However, this shift in opinion may recently have gone too far. There are still cases of ADHD/DAMP and other ESSENCE that have been caused by "pure brain damage" without genetic factors being specifically involved. Furthermore, it is likely that there are many cases where injuries/environmental risk factors and genetic risk factors act in concert to give rise to the neurodevelopmental disorders that manifest as ADHD/DAMP (or indeed other cases of ESSENCE). Nevertheless, it is clear today that many cases previously considered as being due to brain damage were, in fact, more genetically based (Gillberg, 2010; Wilens & Spencer, 2010).

If one seeks to assign percentages to different background factors in ADHD/DAMP, heredity/genes would probably account for about 60% to 70%, and brain damage/environmental biological risks for about 20% to 30%. A relatively large number of cases within the two groups have elements of both heredity and brain damage, albeit one of the factors will be dominant. In around 10% to 15% of cases the cause is still completely unclear (Gillberg & Kadesjö, 2003). Psychosocial factors, in the absence of brain disorders or genetic disposition, do not seem able to cause the fundamental problems of DAMP. However, they do appear to have major, often crucial, significance for the development of secondary problems, particularly in cases of social maladjustment. In extreme cases of depriva- tion, psychosocial factors can themselves lead to "chronic" brain prob- lems that may present with the clinical phenotype of ADHD/DAMP. Interestingly, much of the environmental contribution to the variance of ESSENCE comes from non-shared (rather than shared [i.e., familial]) environment (Lundström et al., 2011).

At the same time, it should be noted that children with attention disor- ders are not necessarily affected by psychosocial factors in the same way as children without ADHD/DAMP. That is not to say that such factors are unimportant in ADHD, but that they may operate differently in such cases as compared with children and teenagers unaffected by ADHD. For instance, children with ADHD may be less aware of parental discord (because of their own inattention problems) than children unaffected by this type of problem, but they may still be very negatively affected by par- ents and others constantly passing negative comments about them.

BOYS AND GIRLS — HOW DIFFERENT ARE THEY?

Boys and girls *are* different, not just in terms of their gender. As improved methods have become available for studying behaviors and abilities, it has become more obvious that boys—as a group—and girls—as a group—dif- fer from the outset of life in many respects, and not merely with regard to such things as external genital characteristics, muscularity, and physical strength. Nevertheless, the variation within the respective genders is vast and the differences between some boys and some girls are very small.

Girls have more rapid social and language development than boys, are better able to concentrate, and are less violent and disruptive than boys of the same age. This is broadly true of all ages before puberty.

On average girls reach puberty 12 to 24 months earlier than boys, a consequence of their central nervous system generally maturing earlier. The implications of this earlier maturation are rarely considered, however.

During childhood boys cause a great deal more problems than girls. It is not simply a matter of them receiving more attention; they have a much higher rate of disorders and behavioral abnormalities of various kinds. The rates of almost all sorts of neuropsychiatric problems are higher among boys than among girls. This goes for most disorders, from ADHD/DAMP and dyslexia through to serious brain disorders. Furthermore, boys are far more accident-prone (not least because of their higher risk of having ADHD) than girls and are thus at increased risk of additional problems.

If girls are so much further ahead in their general maturation and development, and if the rate of disabilities and behavioral disorders is so much lower among them, how can we then expect the same level of school achievements of girls and boys of the same age? An 8-year-old girl ought to have the skills and maturation equivalent to that of a 9- or 10-year-old boy. Yet boys and girls are placed in the same class at the same age. Should they not be put in separate classes, or at least be age-separated within the same class? Why is it not considered reasonable for boys to start school one year later than girls? It is hard to imagine a return to single-sex classes or single-sex schools; there are many negative aspects to the segregation of boys and girls in this manner—including how much duller school would be. Still, there is much to indicate, both in the social and biological development of children, that the majority of boys should start school a year later than the majority of girls.

For example, many boys are not "ready" to read on starting junior school at the age of 6 or 7, let alone at the age of 4 or 5, the age of school start in many countries. Some of these boys do in fact have dyslexia, or other causes of reading and writing difficulties, but for some it is simply a case of "normal slower male maturation." Some boys continue to have difficulty concentrating and sitting still when they are 6 but manage perfectly well at the age of 9. By having boys start school at a slightly later age, one could avoid making a major problem out of this "normal immaturity."

What is the reason for boys' delayed maturation and increased risk of injuries and disorders, primarily those affecting the central nervous system? The causes are numerous and, in part, unknown. The difference in sex chromosome composition and the consequences thereof (e.g., hormonal differences during early brain development) are likely to play the most important role in this, but the mechanisms are still unclear. Girls, with their two X chromosomes, seem to have better "reserves" than boys, who—normally—have only one X chromosome. If disorders or injuries arise in one of their X chromosomes, girls can possibly use the other undamaged chromosome as a backup, which is not the case for boys.

The male sex hormone testosterone appears to inhibit brain development in certain ways. In particular, testosterone seems to have a slowing effect on the development of the left cerebral hemisphere. Slower development of the left cerebral hemisphere ought to result in delayed language—and perhaps also in some aspects of social—development, something that is characteristic of boys. With a relatively immature left cerebral hemisphere, the risk of dyslexia probably increases—a disorder that, as has been mentioned earlier, is much more common among boys. The influence of testosterone on boys also generates greater muscle mass and a higher degree of violent and aggressive behaviors. This leads to an increased risk of disruptive behavior, which, in turn, increases the likelihood of boys receiving more attention, both in a positive and negative sense, for instance in school.

The fact that boys generally have delayed brain maturation means that their brains take longer to become fully developed. It also means that the risk period for incurring damage to the immature brain is longer for boys than it is for girls. Damage to immature nervous tissue has different effects than damage to a fully developed nervous system. Furthermore, boys—for reasons hitherto unknown—are far more prone to risks during pregnancy and childbirth, and sustain brain injuries more frequently than girls during this period.

Another possible reason for girls having *less obvious* ADHD/ESSENCE problems than boys could be the various compensatory mechanisms that would seem to favor girls throughout childhood and adolescence. These would include better early social communication skills, impulse control, and better semantic and episodic memory. As a consequence of these relative advantages, girls (and women) on the whole would be predicted to show fewer (obvious) impairments than boys (and men), and so should be identified and diagnosed less often (or at least much later), even if males and females were afflicted with underlying neurobiological abnormalities at the same rate.

All of the aforementioned factors are independently capable of causing "maturation" differences between boys and girls. Often, however, it is a case of factors having transactional effects, with several playing a role in individual cases.

GENETIC FACTORS

ADHD and DAMP—and many of the other disorders in the ESSENCE group—as studied both in children and adults are very often a result, wholly or partly, of genetic factors (Anckarsäter et al., 2011; Gillberg & Rasmussen, 1982a; Larsson et al., 2013). A father, uncle, grandfather, brother, mother, or sister will have—or will have had—similar problems in 40% to 70% of all cases (Gillberg et al., 1982). Naturally, this is not in itself proof of a genetic cause. Twin and adoption studies, though, indicate that a genetic factor plays a significant role in the majority of cases (Franke et al., 2012). In many studies, however, it has been possible to demonstrate abnormalities in the function of a number of different genes regulating dopamine and noradrenaline function, for instance the gene responsible for the dopamine receptor D4 (Ptácek et al., 2011). The gene for the so-called dopamine transporter protein has also been implicated, but its effect may be modulating rather than directly "causative" (Kebir & Joober, 2011). The function of a particular synapse protein—SNAP-25—is also abnormal in some people with ADHD (Kovács-Nagy et al., 2009). Exactly what it is that is inherited is still unclear in many cases. Dopamine and noradrenaline metabolism abnormalities in the nervous system have so far been able to account for only a minority of the genetic predisposition to ADHD/DAMP. Several other neurotransmitters and nerve growth factors—and genes regulating their metabolism and functioning—might well be involved (Bergman et al., 2011). Some of the synapse and clock genes (e.g., genes regulating melatonin metabolism and functioning) demonstrated to be involved in autism have been implicated in ADHD also (Chaste et al., 2011). In some families there are a whole variety of different ESSENCE problems in different family members; one boy might have ADHD, his brother Asperger syndrome, a sister language disorder, the mother dyslexia, the father ADHD, his brother autism, another of his brothers ADHD, and so forth. Several studies have shown that these are not coincidental findings; instead, the "ESSENCE" problem appears in many guises throughout the family tree, but it is likely that the same set of genes are affected and "responsible" for the whole lot of "behavioral phenotypes" in any given family with this type of history.

Sometimes it is not evident that a similar set of hereditary problems exists. For instance, it could be that motor clumsiness has been passed down through several generations and now manifests in the form of hyperactivity, concentration difficulties, *and* motor difficulties Since the hyperactivity and concentration difficulties are so striking, it is likely that the motor control problems are overlooked and that the link to the problems of previous generations goes unnoticed.

Other times there is no question that *the problem* (i.e., ADHD or DAMP or language disorder per se) "runs in the family" due to a father, uncle, and elder brother having had the same or similar problems. Nevertheless, perhaps their difficulties—for various reasons—have not attracted as much scrutiny as the ones that are the current focus of attention. Hence it can be very difficult to find a reasonable explanation for the presenting problems. Provided one remains persistent and discusses the difficulties from several different perspectives, the predisposing genetic factor should eventually become apparent.

In yet other cases, there is a considerable risk that the genetic factor is missed entirely—for example, if it is only the mother who attends the medical consultation and does not know enough about the father's family, on whose side there is a greater likelihood of a relative having problems similar to those exhibited by the child. The father may have been so ashamed of his own or his family's problems that he has done whatever possible to conceal them. Naturally the mother cannot then be expected to possess sufficient information to determine whether or not a genetic factor is likely to exist.

It is important also to know about the correlation between ADHD/DAMP in childhood and various psychiatric and social problems in adulthood. The genetic factor could go unnoticed if one fails to consider the possibility that certain cases of, for example, social maladjustment, alcoholism, generalized anxiety disorder, atypical depression, bipolar disorder, "personality disorder," and chronic pain syndrome in adulthood might be manifestations of underlying ADHD/DAMP.

POTENTIALLY BRAIN-DAMAGING ENVIRONMENTAL RISK FACTORS

In at least one in three people with ADHD/DAMP, indications of brain-damage risk factors of some kind are present. This is not always equivalent with such factors having actually caused the ADHD, but the negative incident(s) may have contributed to the development of the disorder either in combination with other environmental (including other brain damage) factors or genetic variations/abnormalities of various kinds (Spencer et al., 2007). Risk factors of this kind might well play a role in many other cases of ADHD/DAMP/ESSENCE, and it seems likely that, over the next decade, a number of intricate environment–gene interactions will be shown to be important in neurodevelopmental disorders more generally.

Potential Brain-Damage Risk Factors During Pregnancy

In ADHD/DAMP cases that are caused—either wholly or partially—by brain damage, the cause can usually, although by no means always, be traced to the fetal stage. A variety of factors during pregnancy can precipitate nervous system abnormality and disorders that may later manifest as

ADHD/DAMP symptoms or as disorders within the ESSENCE group. It is hard, though, to single out individual factors. Quite often it is a case of one negative factor leading to another and so on. Many times it is likely to be the case that numerous minor risks and mishaps during pregnancy have collectively prevented the brain from being able to develop under optimal conditions. The term "reduced optimality" is sometimes used to describe such circumstances (Rasmussen et al., 1983). Furthermore, optimality can be reduced to varying extents; the more it is reduced, the greater the risk of neurological and psychiatric consequences (Gillberg, C., & Gillberg, I.C., 1983). To gauge the extent of reduction, it is necessary to draw up a list of a large number of factors (occurrence of high-febrile infections, medication, alcohol, cigarette smoking, high blood pressure, etc.) and to set optimal boundaries for each (e.g., no infection, blood pressure below a certain level). Then, for every factor that does not meet the criteria for optimality, one point is deducted. Once the list has been gone through, all the points are added up to give a total score that indicates by how much optimality has been reduced. The majority of pregnancies have a reduction of zero to four points out of a possible 15 (Kyllerman & Hagberg, 1983). In ADHD/DAMP, two to six points is the norm (Gillberg & Rasmussen, 1982a), and, in certain forms of cerebral palsy, four to eight (Kyllerman, 1983). These results indicate that the risk factors are increased in DAMP, but not as much as in cerebral palsy. However, it is not possible to draw any definite conclusions as to whether the reduced optimality has led to brain injury, or that such brain injury—should it have occurred—is the cause of ADHD/DAMP in that particular case.

Reduced optimality in pregnancy can, of course, be a cause of nervous system damage. Conversely, though, reduced optimality may be indicative of underlying problems in the fetus or the mother. So, for example, psychiatric problems—and hence the associated medication—in the mother could reflect an ADHD syndrome in her own childhood (and one that may or may not be symptomatic now in adult age) and therefore a genetic factor (ADHD) rather than a brain-damage factor (the medication). Naturally, in many cases, it could also be that the different factors interact—a genetic factor (ADHD) in the mother increases the risk of her developing psychiatric problems later in life *and* of her children having ADHD. At the same time, her psychiatric problems lead her to take medication during pregnancy, with the medication *possibly* having a negative impact on the development of the child's brain.

Heavy alcohol consumption and heavy smoking during pregnancy are possibly among the most significant potentially harmful factors in relation to child neurodevelopmental outcomes. There is no doubt that substantial alcohol use and cigarette smoking in pregnancy carry a considerably increased risk of the child having ADHD/DAMP or other disorders within the ESSENCE group, including intellectual developmental disorder, speech and language disorders, and autism (Aronson et al., 1997; Nash et al., 2008). There appears to be a clear correlation between the amount of alcohol consumed in pregnancy and the rate and severity of the disorder in the child. The rate of ESSENCE among schoolchildren would very likely be considerably reduced if all women were able to abstain from alcohol and tobacco smoking during pregnancy. However, the relative contribution of heavy smoking in pregnancy to ADHD in the offspring has yet to be established (Knopik, 2009). It is particularly difficult to disentangle the effects of genetics and environment in this instance. For example, ADHD is highly genetic, meaning that mothers with ADHD will have a much increased risk of having a child with ADHD anyway. It is well established that ADHD is associated with earlier onset and more (and more heavy) smoking than perhaps any other psychiatric disorder, and certainly much above the level in the general population. Smoking in pregnancy is also related to more alcohol use in pregnancy, which in itself increases the risk of ADHD. The poorer the psychosocial setting, the higher is the risk of more alcohol and tobacco use in pregnancy. For all these reasons it is difficult to separate out the individual risks associated with genetics, smoking, alcohol, and psychosocial risk factors, even in well-designed studies. Abuse of certain drugs, including some prescribed ones, in pregnancy also increases the risk of ADHD/DAMP markedly. Thus, while it is relatively straightforward that prenatal exposure to teratogenic substances, including nicotine and alcohol, increases the risk of ADHD and related disorders, studies examining this relationship have usually not investigated the neurobiological pathways involved. However, one study explored the effect of prenatal exposure to cigarettes or alcohol on brain volume in children with ADHD and typically developing controls (de Zeeuw et al., 2012). Children with ADHD who had been exposed in utero to either substance were matched to children with and without ADHD who had not been. For prenatal exposure to both smoking and alcohol, the authors found a significant gradient where subjects with ADHD who had been exposed had the smallest brain volumes and unexposed controls had the largest, with intermediate volumes for unexposed subjects with ADHD. The effect was most significant for the cerebellum.

As has already been mentioned, use of medication in pregnancy can cause problems of the ESSENCE type in individual cases. In these instances it is generally a case of medication having been taken over a long period of time rather than on just one or two occasions.

Extremely or very premature birth—for example, after 24 to 32 weeks instead of 40—increases the risk of brain injury and ADHD/DAMP greatly (Scott et al., 2012). Only 20 years ago it was rare for extremely premature children to survive into school age. This is no longer the case, and hence the causal panorama of ADHD/DAMP has changed; premature birth is nowadays an important and increasingly prevalent risk factor for ADHD/DAMP. Preterm and early-term birth increases the risk of ADHD by increasing degrees of immaturity. This effect does not appear to be explained by genetic, perinatal, or socioeconomic factors, but socioeconomic factors do *modify* the risk of ADHD in moderately preterm births (Lindström et al., 2011).

A large number of pregnancy factors that have a negative influence on the development of the placenta increase the child's risk of ADHD/DAMP and other ESSENCE. These include diabetes, heart and kidney disease, chronic infections, and maternal toxemia (high blood pressure, proteinuria, and generalized swelling/edema). If placental function deteriorates, there is an increased risk of the child being born with poor reserves of fat and starch. Consequently there is a major risk that the child will be unable to cope with the relative starvation of the neonatal stage, and that bouts of low blood sugar and low nerve sugar levels will occur. Low nerve sugar levels carry an impending risk of permanent damage. Brain injuries incurred in this manner can be prevented to a certain extent through early additional feeding for children weighing less than expected relative to the length of pregnancy.

Potential Brain-Damage Risk Factors Around the Time of Child's Birth

When it was the catch-term for virtually all disorders within the ESSENCE group, "MBD" was generally considered to be caused by injury at or around the time of birth (and was often thought of as "minimal brain *damage*"). Most of the systematic research performed in the area suggests that this was an incorrect assumption in many cases (Gillberg & Rasmussen, 1982b; Rutter, 1982). Injuries to the child's nervous system sustained around the actual delivery have a relatively small impact on the overall panorama of risk for ADHD/DAMP or other ESSENCE. This does not mean that ADHD/DAMP cannot arise as a result of birth injuries, merely that such injuries are not particularly common causes. However, asphyxia—intrapartal and extrauterine—, with ensuing hypoxic ischemic encephalopathy (HIE) probably does play a role as an important epidemiological risk factor in the etiology of ADHD/DAMP and other ESSENCE, accounting for more of the variance than currently assumed (Getahun et al., 2013, Lindström et al., 2006). Asphyxia as an isolated problem has relatively little significance as far as the occurrence of ADHD/DAMP is concerned. However, in cases where asphyxia is only the culmination of negative development that has persisted throughout the entire pregnancy, lack of oxygen can prove the "final straw."

Traumatic births are also often preceded by conditions of "reduced optimality" in pregnancy. In such cases it can sometimes be difficult to determine which factor has caused the brain injury.

Cerebral hemorrhage and cerebral cysts with or without a history of cerebral hemorrhage, often followed by seizures during the neonatal stage and pronounced sucking difficulties later on, is a rare but important cause of subsequent ADHD/DAMP problems (Millichap, 1997; Wester et al., 2001).

Some studies indicate that breech delivery increases the risk of ADHD/DAMP later in life (Fianu & Joelsson, 1979). However, the breech position itself could be an indication of abnormal development, and the delivery circumstances may have little or no correlation with the DAMP problems. A number of studies, though, suggest that children in the breech position who were delivered via cesarean section have a markedly lower rate of ADHD/DAMP in school age compared with breech children who were delivered "normally."

Brain-Damage Risk Factors During the First Years of Life

Brain infections and inflammation during the first two or three years of life are sometimes followed by ADHD/DAMP and other problems of the ESSENCE type. This is rare, however, and in a group of 100 children with DAMP there is unlikely to be a single child with such a background. Nevertheless, in a select few cases, encephalitis following a bout of measles, mumps, chicken pox, whooping cough, or herpes infection will be the cause of ADHD/DAMP. It is also probable that Lyme disease resulting from a tick bite can give rise to symptoms similar to those encountered in ADHD/DAMP and other ESSENCE (Fallon et al., 1998).

Treatments for childhood cancer, including irradiation of the brain, and a variety of chemotherapies increase the risk of later attentional problems in the child, particularly the types of problems typically seen in ADHD of the inattentive subtype (Parsay et al., 2011). One in five to in four children treated with methotrexate for acute leukemia develop problems of the ESSENCE type. Folate pathway polymorphisms appear to be playing a crucial role in some cases of ADHD developing after such malignancies (Kamdar et al., 2011).

Concussion, in general, appears to have little bearing on the development of ADHD/DAMP and other ESSENCE. However, there is some uncertainty regarding this ever since reports on the delayed effects of concussion, including ADHD/DAMP symptoms, emerged a few years ago (Chan, 2002; Smits et al., 2009). On the other hand, it must be remembered that the risk of children with ADHD/DAMP suffering concussion is higher than normal, which could give the impression of a causal link between concussion and ADHD/DAMP.

Lead poisoning, or lead exposure of a more moderate nature, can manifest as ADHD/DAMP symptoms (Thapar et al., 2012). Lead is unlikely to be a common cause of ADHD/DAMP in Sweden but could be in certain mining areas of England, for example, meaning that its relative contribution to etiological variance in ADHD is possibly highly variable. Mercury can also have negative effects on brain function, manifesting as a number of symptoms typical of ADHD (Weihe et al., 2003).

Serious traumatic brain injuries are often followed by concentration difficulties, short-term memory problems, fluctuating wakefulness, irritability, and abnormal sleep patterns. All of these symptoms are also typical of ADHD/DAMP (Karver et al., 2012). Generally, though, there will be other neurological symptoms that make the connection to the brain injury more likely. In certain cases of serious traumatic brain injury, one needs to be open to the possibility that the ADHD/DAMP problems may have been present prior to the brain injury occurring.

OTHER FACTORS POSSIBLY CONTRIBUTING TO THE ETIOLOGICAL VARIANCE IN ADHD

Reduction of artificial colorants in food has been shown to decrease ADHD-type symptoms under randomized controlled conditions (Egger et al., 1985). The effect that such colorants might have on underlying brain dysfunction in ADHD or whether they can themselves cause or contribute to brain dysfunction is currently not understood.

Omega-3/Omega-6 supplementation has been shown to have positive effects on ADHD symptoms in a subgroup of all those affected, and clinical improvement was associated with plasma fatty acid concentration change, supporting the notion that reduced levels of fatty acids in the organism could be a factor contributing to ADHD symptomatology in the population (Johnson et al., 2009, 2012).

Low levels of vitamin D have been increasingly noted in young children spending a lot of their time indoors rather than out of doors (McCurdy et al., 2010). Particularly low levels of vitamin D were recently found in ADHD in a Swedish study (Humble, 2010). It is possible that low levels of vitamin D increase the risk of a number of neurodevelopmental disorders (Kočovská et al., 2012), but there is a need for much more research in the field before more definitive conclusions can be drawn regarding the role of vitamin D in ADHD, ASD, and other disorders within the ESSENCE group.

The influence of diets on children's behavior and behavioral problems has only recently been the subject of systematic research attention. While very few firm conclusions can be drawn at this stage, one has to assume that diets "for" (or rather "against") ADHD will become much more discussed in the very near future (Millichap & Yee, 2012).

EEG FINDINGS

In approximately onethird of ADHD cases and in twothirds of DAMP cases (and in at least half of all ESSENCE cases), EEG results are abnormal (Matousek 1983). This includes all types of abnormalities, from those that are probably fairly benign to those that reflect severe brain disorders.

The most common type of abnormality, and the one that is most characteristic of ADHD/DAMP, is "moderate nonspecific abnormality" (Gillberg et al., 1984). This means that there is a markedly increased amount of slow EEG activity, suggestive of what is seen in considerably younger children, but also encountered in cases of generalized brain damage.

Some children with ADHD/DAMP exhibit distinct epileptogenic EEG activity. Outbursts, volatility, or generally impaired mental functioning can occur without warning in such cases. Sometimes a direct chronological correlation can be demonstrated between the occurrence of such problems and the sudden onset of epileptiform EEG activity. Certain children with these types of problems may benefit from treatment with antiepileptic medication. The same goes for a small group of children with severe DAMP who display epileptogenic EEG activity only in connection with trigger factors of various kinds, such as stimulation from flickering lights, hyperventilation, or decreased wakefulness.

Many children with ADHD/DAMP have mild EEG abnormalities similar to those occasionally seen in control subjects without any diagnosed problems. Upon closer analysis of the children in the control group who have EEG abnormalities, it quite often transpires that some of them have mild DAMP-like difficulties. In other words, it is possible for children and adolescents who are entirely "normal" to exhibit mild EEG abnormalities. Admittedly, their behavior is within the normal spectrum, but it is often redolent of what is seen, albeit in more pronounced form, in DAMP. It is essential that all children and adolescents with more severe forms of ADHD/DAMP have an EEG, chiefly to detect certain forms of epilepsy that have few overt symptoms. Such forms of epilepsy can be treated effectively and may sometimes also result in a complete resolution of DAMP symptoms. An EEG is not, however, necessary for making a diagnosis of ADHD/DAMP.

NEUROIMAGING FINDINGS

Long-term follow-up of children with ADHD using MRI scans has shown that brain volume is somewhat reduced and that the frontal lobes, cerebellum, parts of the corpus callosum, and basal ganglia (corpus striatum) are slightly smaller than in same-age peers without ADHD. The volume reduction remains throughout puberty with no signs of "maturation" or "catch-up." Other studies, in which children with ADHD have been compared with their siblings, indicate a genetic predisposition to slightly smaller brain size, and also that the cerebellum is specifically affected in ADHD. Approximately one in four children with DAMP have some clear structural brain abnormality that can be depicted on brain scans. These abnormalities can be located in a number of regions of the brain, but usually in the frontal and parietal lobes. No DAMP-specific pattern has been detected, however. There are abnormalities in terms of the normal asymmetrical development of the anterior portions of the brain.

There are clear timing deficits in ADHD. A meta-regression analysis of 11 fMRI studies showed that right dorsolateral prefrontal cortex activation was reduced in previously unmedicated patients but normal in patients receiving long-term stimulants relative to controls, suggesting potential normalization effects on the function of this prefrontal region with long-term psychostimulant treatment (Hart et al., 2012).

Results from network-based statistical analyses of fMRI findings have isolated two brain network regions (one frontal amygdala-occipital and another frontal temporal-occipital) between which interregional connectivity may be significantly altered in ADHD (Cocchi et al., 2012). The findings highlight the importance of extending the conceptualization of ADHD beyond segregated frontostriatal alterations.

Measurement of cerebral blood flow via single photon emission computed tomography (SPECT) scanning often reveals patches of reduced blood flow in the brain. Reduced cerebral blood flow generally reflects reduced nerve function (Di Tommaso, 2012).

Using another method of cerebral blood flow measurement, positron emission tomography (PET) imaging, it has been possible, for example in Danish studies, to demonstrate abnormalities located centrally in the brain (in the corpus striatum, among other regions) of children with ADHD/DAMP.

All these results have major theoretical significance. However, in the majority of cases, the aforementioned scans have no role to play in the examination of a child or teenager with ADHD/DAMP. Locating the brain injuries and functional changes that may lie at the root of the DAMP symptoms does not currently provide any indication—in normal cases—that the treatment strategy should change. If the scan has no bearing on either treatment or continued investigation, there are generally no grounds for performing it. In a select few cases, though, there may be psychological indications. Should suspicion of another neurological disorder arise, there is a case for carrying out one or more of the aforementioned neuroimaging scans.

BRAIN STEM AUDIOMETRY ABNORMALITIES AND OTHER AUDITORY TRACT PROBLEMS IN ADHD AND RELATED DISORDERS

The results of brainstem audiometry are abnormal in some children with ADHD/DAMP/other ESSENCE and, perhaps particularly, in children with the combination of ADHD and epilepsy (Major, 2011; Rosenhall et al., 2003). Such abnormalities are indicative of disorders affecting central stimuli processing centers—in, among other areas, the brainstem— and may support the theory regarding impaired automatization skills.

The positive effect of white noise in ADHD (Söderlund et al., 2007) may be partly accounted for by brainstem dysfunction and stochastic resonance (i.e., the phenomenon that moderate noise facilitates cognitive performance). It is suggested that noise in the environment introduces internal noise into the neural system by way of the perceptual system. This noise induces stochastic resonance in the neurotransmitter systems and makes this noise beneficial for cognitive performance. In particular, the peak of the stochastic resonance curve depends on the dopamine level, so that participants with low dopamine levels (i.e., many with ADHD) require more noise for optimal cognitive performance compared to controls.

CONDITIONS THAT CAN MANIFEST AS ADHD/DAMP AND OTHER ESSENCE

A smaller group of children with DAMP have underlying specific—and nowadays diagnosable—chromosomal or DNA content abnormalities. In the future it will probably be possible to diagnose many more cases of ADHD/ DAMP using DNA methods. To date, of the disorders that are diagnosable by chromosomal or DNA analysis, it is mainly sex chromosome abnormalities (an extra X or Y chromosome in boys, an X chromosome short in girls), fragile X chromosome, and certain genetic conditions with particular behavioral profiles (e.g., 22q11 deletion syndrome ["CATCH-22"], Williams syndrome, and Prader-Willi syndrome) that often produce ADHD symptoms.

Diseases and disorders such as hypomelanosis of Ito, neurofibromatosis, and tuberous sclerosis also frequently generate ADHD/DAMP symptoms, but there is currently no simple blood test for these that could help
form the basis for diagnosis.

In different forms of goiter (diseases of the thyroid gland)—with low
metabolism (hypothyroidism) or increased metabolism (hyperthyroid-
ism)—it is possible for ADHD/DAMP symptoms to dominate completely
before other symptoms come to the fore. Some studies have suggested that
people with ADHD have a resistance to thyroid hormone, whereas other
studies indicate that a possible correlation is tenuous. Metabolic disorders
must, however, always be considered in cases of ADHD, especially if the
symptoms have not been apparent from the first years of life.

ALLERGIES

Over the past 20 years there have been categorical claims of a strong correlation between allergy and ADHD. It now seems as though these must
be regarded as a greatly modified version of the truth. In a subgroup of
children with ADHD, perhaps particularly within the left-handed group,
allergies do occur that, if not treated satisfactorily, can result in deteriora-
tion, not least in terms of the child's behavior.

Several independent and carefully controlled studies indicate that the
elimination of certain foods from the diet can lead to significant improvement in conduct disorders in certain children with proven allergies. In
some studies it has been a case of eliminating milk and strong coloring
agents, in others of eliminating various foods that the child has appeared
unable to tolerate (Carter et al., 1993; Egger et al., 1985; Rucklidge
et al., 2011).

It is difficult to draw any general conclusions on the basis of the studies that have been carried out. However, a fair interpretation would be for
children with a strong genetic predisposition to allergy, or actual allergy
symptoms, to be tried on an elimination diet if they show signs of ADHD/
DAMP.

IS THERE A CORRELATION WITH HANDEDNESS?

Within all groups of people with brain injuries, there is an increased prevalence of left-handedness or "non-right-handedness." This is a natural consequence of the fact that the majority of all people (90% to 95%) are genetically intended to be predominantly right-handed and that a minority (5% to 10%) are intended to be left-handed. Brain injuries—when they occur—are either bilateral or unilateral. Unilateral injuries affect the left and right cerebral hemispheres with equal frequency. The injury has no preference, so to speak. In other words, half of the time the left cerebral hemisphere, which controls the movements of the right hand, is affected, and half of the time the right cerebral hemisphere, which dictates the movements of the left hand, is affected.

Given that the right hand is almost always the one that a child is genetically predestined to prefer, a relatively large number of those who sustain unilateral brain injuries will switch from being right-handed to being left-handed. Moreover, given that the left hand is so seldom the one that a child is predestined to prefer, relatively few of those who suffer unilateral brain injuries will switch from being left-handed to being right-handed. Essentially what this means is that, of those who are manifestly left-handed, a greater relative proportion have this preference as a result of brain injury, compared with the corresponding proportion of those who are manifestly right-handed.

Approximately 15% of children with DAMP are left-handed, and around another 15% are non-right-handed (left-handed or ambidextrous) (Rasmussen et al., 1983). This means that, in total, nearly one in three children in a DAMP group are non-right-handed, compared with roughly one in eight in a group of children who do not have DAMP. At the same time, the figures also show that the vast majority of all people with DAMP are "normally" right-handed. There is continued debate as to whether left-handedness is more common in ADHD generally than in the general population. However, there is suggestive evidence that "non-right-handedness" (i.e., left-handedness or ambidexterity) is considerably more common in young children with inattention, distractibility, and language disorder than in children without such symptoms in the general population (Rodriguez & Waldenström, 2008).

SOCIAL FACTORS

"Social factors" is an extremely vague term, one that usually crops up in books on psychiatric problems without ever actually being defined. Social factors encompass everything from "society at large" to one's immediate environment, peers, friends, relatives, and family.

Social factors are seldom or never clear-cut; for example, they frequently have both bioenvironmental and genetic aspects. An example of this is parental alcoholism, a background factor that has a major influence on the development of psychiatric problems in children, and one that is very often regarded as a predominantly social—or possibly, to use an even vaguer term, psychosocial—factor. However, alcoholism in a parent also has potential genetic significance. It is known that even children who were given up for adoption early in life, and who have biological parents who are alcoholics and adoptive parents who are not, run an increased risk of falling victim to alcohol abuse themselves. Maternal alcoholism in pregnancy also carries major risks for the fetus and, in this context, alcohol too can be considered a bioenvironmental toxin. Social factors, such as lack of care and supervision, can lead to a heightened risk of accidents that may, for instance, affect the head and brain, thereby increasing the risk of injuries to the central nervous system. Conversely, children with brain disorders are at increased risk of "attracting" a multitude of unfavorable social factors, including destructive gangs, bullying "friends," and arguing parents. This short list of examples illustrates how tricky it is to isolate specific social/psychosocial factors. It is remarkable, in fact, how common it is for terms such as "social factors"—and "social causes" in particular—to be taken for granted without any attempt to analyze them, let alone define them. This chapter is no shining exception to the rule, but it is important to be aware that social factors are nearly always ambiguous and thus difficult to pronounce on definitively.

There is much to suggest that children's mental health—generally speaking—has deteriorated over the past 50 years, at least in the Western world. At the same time, their social circumstances—materially speaking—have improved markedly. Hence socioeconomic factors cannot easily be singled out as the root cause of why today's children have a far higher rate of mental disorders than previous generations (Richards, 2013).

Virtually all studies of children's mental health, however, point to a strong correlation between mental disorder and "family dysfunction." Over the past 50 years the family and its role has changed considerably. Divorce was relatively uncommon in the 1950s; nowadays it is the norm rather than the exception. Children today often live with a large number of adults who are expected to play some part in their upbringing: mother; father; stepfather; stepmother; stepfather number two; stepmother number two; kindergarten head; kindergarten teachers number one, two, three, four, five; youth recreation leader; schoolteachers; and so forth. While it used to be taken for granted that a child's upbringing was the parents' role, it is par for the course these days for a great number of other people to be involved. If the family is not functioning well in such a situation, there is a major risk of the child having no one who truly cares about his or her well-being. All people need, in the words of Alice Miller, to be "seen." Furthermore, all children need to be especially important to someone. In today's society it is probably not uncommon for children to fall somewhere in between; no one assumes primary responsibility for the individual child's development and upbringing.

Children with ADHD/DAMP are no exception when it comes to the negative influence of certain social factors. On average they come from a somewhat lower social group than children in general. The reason for this is unknown, but a number of factors could possibly be acting collectively. Parents of children with DAMP quite often have similar problems themselves and are consequently hampered—due to, among other things, concentration and learning problems of their own—in developing their full potential or going far in their careers. Naturally, having a child with difficulties can in itself also contribute to parents having neither the time nor energy to spare to devote to their own education or careers. Social problems contribute heavily to the development of psychiatric problems, primarily acting-out behaviors (including antisocial, aggressive, and violent behavior), in children with ADHD/DAMP. However, it is important to state that children with ADHD/DAMP from lower social groups fare as well as those from higher ones, provided that no particularly adverse psychosocial conditions are present. It is relevant also to mention that siblings of children with DAMP often do well, assuming that they themselves do not have DAMP.

THE ROLE OF FAMILY

The family's role is very important in cases of ADHD/DAMP, not just because of the condition itself, but because a "well-functioning" family—whatever that is—has a major bearing on the development of everyone's mental well-being. Some studies indicate that children with attention disorders may actually be even *less* negatively affected than other children by a dysfunctional family (Breslau, 1990). It would appear that the concentration and attention impairments also pertain to the child's ability to register and reflect on negative parental interaction. If, on the other hand, the parents constantly—and specifically—direct their anger toward the child, this contributes to the latter developing low self-esteem or antisocial behavior.

Several studies show that children with ADHD/DAMP and their parents affect one another in a complex fashion (Richards, 2013). First and foremost, the child's problems result in the mother, father, and siblings acquiring negative attitudes—at least until the child receives a diagnosis, or they gain a deeper understanding of the child's fundamental difficulties. They yell at and find fault with the child and act—sometimes excessively so, sometimes justifiably—in a controlling manner. If the child's abnormal behavior is temporarily normalized, for example with the aid of stimulant medication, the behaviors and attitudes of the mother and siblings are normalized as well. This demonstrates to some extent the chicken-and-egg nature of the negative interaction between the child with DAMP and the rest of the family.

The negative words and nagging lead to an escalation of conduct disorders in the child with ADHD/DAMP (Gillberg, I.C., & Gillberg, C., 1983;

Woodward et al., 1998). In turn, this further increases negative interactions with other family members, who grow increasingly frustrated and resort to threats and raising their voice more and more. Clearly, this does nothing to improve the child's situation and a vicious circle is started. This circle can have very negative consequences, even in families that are warm and fundamentally loving. The most damaging consequences naturally occur in a harsh, cold, or disengaged family environment where family members break the frosty atmosphere only to scold, shout, or hit.

If the family is not given help to understand the child's fundamental difficulties, there is an impending risk that the vicious circle is set in motion prior to school age.

THE ROLE OF SCHOOLS AND SCHOOLING

An "ignorant" school generally reacts in a similar way to that of parents and siblings. If teachers and classmates believe that all the child's problems could be eradicated if only he or she "pulled himself or herself together," they start—often without being aware of it—a bullying process. Moreover, if classmates do not understand that the child's trying behavior is a manifestation of a genuine disorder, they will not want to play with him or her. Likewise, no teacher finds it enjoyable trying to teach someone who is unreceptive.

For the child with ADHD/DAMP, school is often the final straw. The child may possibly have a sympathetic teacher in the first years of primary school, but in later years there is rarely anyone who truly understands what is wrong. By this point, all of the secondary problems, reading and writing difficulties, depression, and conduct disorders are in full bloom, and it becomes increasingly hard to discern the vulnerable child with all of his or her hidden difficulties in the midst of these other problems. The same scenario also occurs at sixth-form college; at university, however, staff is often better informed.

Reading and writing difficulties in particular, including the specific difficulties referred to as dyslexia, constitute a very negative factor for

the majority of children with DAMP. In many places, schools still possess inadequate knowledge about how best such difficulties should be
addressed and treated. By misunderstanding these difficulties and view-
ing them as laziness, stupidity, or over ambition (in those who struggle
intensely to overcome them), schools contribute to low self-esteem and
depression—and, in the long run, to acting-out behavior.

Well-conducted studies have shown, among other things, that school
tasks need to be made "interesting" in order for children with ADHD—even
if they are on medication (see Chapter 12)—to be able to solve/complete
them. It is not easy to know how one is supposed to capture the interest of
a pupil with ADHD if one is unaware that the child has extreme concentration difficulties and is distracted by irrelevant stimuli. These factors alone
are a clear reason why all teachers must be educated about ADHD.

PSYCHOLOGICAL FACTORS

Psychological factors refer to how individuals perceive themselves, their
difficulties, and their surroundings. A child who, from a very young age,
hears, "Look out! Watch yourself! Mind the table! Don't tug at the table-
cloth! You're not allowed there! Stop! I'm going crazy! Can't you ever keep
still? Now calm down! Don't get up! Concentrate on what you're doing!
Don't move! Careful of your brother! Close your mouth! Hurry up! Stop
daydreaming and listen to me! Pull yourself together for once! I know you
could if you'd just put your mind to it! Clumsy clod! We won't have time if
you don't get a move on!" and a thousand other, often far worse, things—
generally uttered in an irritated or angry tone, or even a bawling rage—is
scarcely likely to develop a positive self-image.

It is not only parents and siblings who complain or grow resigned. Peers
and subsequently teachers and other school staff continue to bombard the
child with complaints.

From early in life, many children with ADHD/DAMP feel different and
inadequate. They do not have the ability to meet the expectations, whether
explicit or implicit, at home or the demands of peers and teachers at

preschool/school. A frequent consequence of this is negative self-perception and a general sense of stupidity, a conviction of not being good enough, of there being no point in even trying, since failure is practically guaranteed. The child says, "I can't" without daring to try. Even more commonly heard is, "I don't want to," which most of the time essentially means, "I don't think I'm able to." In these cases, the road to depression is easy to foresee.

Certain children with ADHD/DAMP have a naïve lack of awareness of their difficulties and come across, at least initially, as blithely overestimating their own ability. Some of these children gradually become increasingly aware of their difficulties—and thus generally both sad and angry. Others never veer from their early discernible cheerful demeanor and will trivialize their difficulties, often throughout their whole lives. It is primarily a smaller group within the group with clearly defined ADHD problems, as well as some with borderline intelligence, who tend to develop in this way.

Some children within the ADHD/DAMP group, often those who are extremely hyperactive, are so inattentive that nothing seems to "sink in," with "everything going in one ear and out the other." It is as though they fail to notice everyone complaining about them. Nor do they appear to react if their parents are arguing with one another. Paradoxically enough, some children with such severe ADHD/DAMP problems can be less sensitive than other children to heated family arguments and chronic discord.

CONCLUDING REMARKS

ADHD/DAMP and other ESSENCE are often caused by genetic factors, more rarely by brain damage/dysfunction sustained during early development, and, perhaps quite commonly, by an interaction of the two. Social factors, particularly within the family and school, contribute in many cases to the development of some additional mental/psychiatric disorders, but probably not to the "ADHD per se." For children with ADHD/DAMP and other ESSENCE to achieve as good a quality of life as possible, parents, siblings, peers, and teachers must know about the child's difficulties so that they can help rather than hinder matters.

REFERENCES

Anckarsäter, H., Lundström, S., Kollberg, L., Kerekes, N., Palm, C., Carlström, E., et al. (2011). The Child and Adolescent Twin Study in Sweden (CATSS). *Twin Research and Human Genetics, 14,* 495–508.

Aronson, M., Hagberg, B., & Gillberg, C. (1997). Attention deficits and autistic spectrum problems in children exposed to alcohol during gestation: a follow-up study. *Developmental Medicine and Child Neurology, 39,* 583–587.

Bergman, O., Westberg, L., Lichtenstein, P., Eriksson, E., & Larsson, H. (2011). Study on the possible association of brain-derived neurotrophic factor polymorphism with the developmental course of symptoms of attention deficit and hyperactivity. *International Journal of Neuropsychopharmacology, 14,* 1367–1376.

Breslau, N. (1990). Does brain dysfunction increased children's vulnerability to environmental stress? *Archives of General Psychiatry, 47,* 15–20.

Carter, C.M., Urbanowicz, M., Hemsley, R., Mantilla, L., Strobel, S., Graham, P.J., et al. (1993). Effects of a few food diet in attention deficit disorder. *Archives of Disease in Childhood, 69,* 564–568.

Chan, R.C. (2002). Attentional deficits in patients with persisting postconcussive complaints: a general deficit or specific component deficit? *Journal of Clinical and Experimental Neuropsychology, 24,* 1081–1093.

Chaste, P., Clement, N., Botros, H.G., Guillaume, J.L., Konyukh, M., Pagan, C., et al. (2011). Genetic variations of the melatonin pathway in patients with attention-deficit and hyperactivity disorders. *Journal of Pineal Research, 51,* 394–399.

Cocchi, L., Bramati, I.E., Zalesky, A., Furukawa, E., Fontenelle, L.F., Moll, J., et al. (2012). Altered functional brain connectivity in a non-clinical sample of young adults with attention-deficit/hyperactivity disorder. *Journal of Neuroscience, 32,* 17753–17761.

de Zeeuw, P., Zwart, F., Schrama, R., van Engeland, H., & Durston, S. (2012). Prenatal exposure to cigarette smoke or alcohol and cerebellum volume in attention-deficit/hyperactivity disorder and typical development. *Translational Psychiatry, 2,* e84.

Di Tommaso, M.C. (2012). A comparative study of bipolar disorder and attention deficit hyperactivity disorder through the measurement of regional cerebral blood flow. *Journal of Biological Regulators and Homeostatic Agents, 26,* 1–6.

Egger, J., Carter, C.M., Graham, P.J., Gumley, D., & Soothill, J.F. (1985). Controlled trial of oligoantigenic treatment in the hyperkinetic syndrome. *Lancet, 1,* 540–545.

Fallon, B.A., Kochevar, J.M., Gaito, A., & Nields, J.A. (1998). The under diagnosis of neuropsychiatric Lyme disease in children and adults. *Psychiatric Clinics of North America, 21,* 693–703.

Fianu, S., & Joelsson, I. (1979). Minimal brain dysfunction in children born in breech presentation. *Acta Obstetricia et Gynecologica Scandinavica, 58,* 295–299.

Franke, B., Faraone, S.V., Asherson, P., Buitelaar, J., Bau, C.H., Ramos-Quiroga, J.A., et al. (2012). The genetics of attention deficit/hyperactivity disorder in adults, a review. *Molecular Psychiatry, 17,* 960–987.

Getahun, D., Rhoads, G.G., Demissie, K., Lu, S.E., Quinn, V.P., Fassett, M.J. et al. (2013) In utero exposure to ischemic-hypoxic conditions and attention-deficit/hyperactivity disorder. *Pediatrics, 131,* e53-61. Gillberg, C. (2010). The ESSENCE in child psychiatry: early symptomatic syndromes eliciting neurodevelopmental clinical examinations. *Research in Developmental Disabilities, 31,* 1543–1551.

Gillberg, C., & Gillberg, I.C. (1983). Infantile autism: a total population study of reduced optimality in the pre-, peri-, and neonatal period. *Journal of Autism and Developmental Disorders, 13,* 153–166.

Gillberg, C., & Kadesjö, B. (2003). Why bother about clumsiness? The implications of having developmental coordination disorder (DCD). *Neural Plasticity, 10,* 59–68.

Gillberg, C., & Rasmussen, P. (1982a). Perceptual, motor and attentional deficits in seven-year-old children: background factors. *Developmental Medicine and Child Neurology, 24,* 752–770.

Gillberg, C., & Rasmussen, P. (1982b). [A study in Gothenburg: minimal brain dysfunction in 6–7-year-old children can be traced by simple diagnostic aids]. *Läkartidningen, 79,* 4413–4414, 4419.

Gillberg, C., Matousek, M., Petersén, I., & Rasmussen, P. (1984). Perceptual, motor and attentional deficits in seven-year-old children. Electroencephalographic aspects. *Acta Paedopsychiatrica, 50,* 243–253.

Gillberg, C., Rasmussen, P., Carlström, G., Svenson, B., & Waldenström, E. (1982). Perceptual, motor and attentional deficits in six-year-old children. Epidemiological aspects. *Journal of Child Psychology and Psychiatry, 23,* 131–144.

Gillberg, I.C., & Gillberg, C. (1983). Three-year follow-up at age 10 of children with minor neurodevelopmental disorders. I: Behavioural problems. *Developmental Medicine and Child Neurology, 25,* 438–449.

Hart, H., Radua, J., Mataix-Cols, D., & Rubia, K. (2012). Meta-analysis of fMRI studies of timing in attention-deficit hyperactivity disorder (ADHD). *Neuroscience and Biobehavioral Reviews, 36,* 2248–2256.

Humble, M.B. (2010). Vitamin D, light and mental health. *Journal of Photochemistry and Photobiology, 101,* 142–149.

Johnson, M., Östlund, S., Fransson, G., Kadesjö, B., & Gillberg, C. (2009). Omega-3/omega-6 fatty acids for attention deficit hyperactivity disorder: a randomized placebo-controlled trial in children and adolescents. *Journal of Attention Disorders, 12,* 394–401.

Johnson, M., Månsson, J.E., Östlund, S., Fransson, G., Areskoug, B., Hjalmarsson, K., et al. (2012). Fatty acids in ADHD: plasma profiles in a placebo-controlled study of omega 3/6 fatty acids in children and adolescents. *Attention Deficit and Hyperactivity Disorders, 4,* 199–204.

Kamdar, K.Y., Krull, K.R., El-Zein, R.A., Brouwers, P., Potter, B.S., Harris, L.L., et al. (2011). Folate pathway polymorphisms predict deficits in attention and processing speed after childhood leukemia therapy. *Pediatric Blood & Cancer, 57,* 454–460.

Karver, C.L., Wade, S.L., Cassedy, A., Taylor, H.G., Stancin, T., Yeates, K.O., et al. (2012). Age at injury and long-term behavior problems after traumatic brain injury in young children. *Rehabilitation Psychology, 57,* 256–265.

Kebir, O., & Joober, R. (2011). Neuropsychological endophenotypes in attention-deficit/hyperactivity disorder: a review of genetic association studies. *European Archives of Psychiatry and Clinical Neuroscience, 261,* 583–594.

Kočovská, E., Fernell, E., Billstedt, E., Minnis, H., & Gillberg, C. (2012). Vitamin D and autism: clinical review. *Research in Developmental Disabilities, 33*, 1541–1550.

Kovács-Nagy, R., Hu, J., Rónai, Z., & Sasvári-Székely, M. (2009). SNAP-25: a novel candidate gene in psychiatric genetics. *Neuropsychopharmacologia Hungarica, 11*, 89–94.

Knopik, V.S. (2009). Maternal smoking during pregnancy and child outcomes: real or spurious effect? *Developmental Neuropsychology, 34*, 1–36.

Kyllerman, M. (1983). Reduced optimality in pre- and perinatal conditions in dyskinetic cerebral palsy—distribution and comparison to controls. *Neuropediatrics, 14*, 29–36.

Kyllerman, M., & Hagberg, G. (1983). Reduced optimality in pre- and perinatal conditions in a Swedish newborn population. *Neuropediatrics, 14*, 37–42.

Larsson, H., Asherson, P., Chang, Z., Ljung, T., Friedrichs, B., Larsson, J.O., et al. (2013). Genetic and environmental influences on adult attention deficit hyperactivity disorder symptoms: a large Swedish population-based study of twins. *Psychological Medicine, 43*, 197–207.

Lindström, K., Lindblad, F., & Hjern, A. (2011). Preterm birth and attention-deficit/ hyperactivity disorder in schoolchildren. *Pediatrics, 127*, 858–865.

Lindström, K., Lagerroos, P., Gillberg, C., & Fernell, E. (2006). Teenage outcome after being born at term with moderate neonatal encephalopathy. *Pediatric Neurology, 35*, 268–274.

Lundström, S., Chang, Z., Kerekes, N., Gumpert, C.H., Råstam, M., Gillberg, C., et al. (2011). Autistic-like traits and their association with mental health problems in two nationwide twin cohorts of children and adults. *Psychological Medicine, 41*, 2423–2433.

Major, Z.Z. (2011). Combined evoked potentials in co-occurring attention deficit hyperactivity disorder and epilepsy. *Ideggyógyászati szemle, 64*, 248–256.

Makris, N., Biederman, J., Monuteaux, M.C., & Seidman, L.J. (2009). Towards conceptualizing a neural systems-based anatomy of attention-deficit/hyperactivity disorder. *Developmental Neuroscience, 31*, 36–49.

Matousek, M. (1983). EEG vigilance profile as a supplement of psychiatric data. *Neuropsychobiology, 9*, 250–253.

McCurdy, L.E., Winterbottom, K.E., Mehta, S.S., & Roberts, J.R. (2010). Using nature and outdoor activity to improve children's health. *Current Problems in Pediatric and Adolescent Health Care, 40*, 102–117.

Millichap, J.G. (1997). Encephalitis virus and attention deficit hyperactivity disorder. *Journal of the Royal Society of Medicine, 90*, 709–710.

Millichap, J.G., & Yee, M.M. (2012). The diet factor in attention-deficit/hyperactivity disorder. *Pediatrics, 129*, 330–337.

Nash, K., Sheard, E., Rovet, J., & Koren, G. (2008). Understanding fetal alcohol spectrum disorders (FASDs): toward identification of a behavioral phenotype. *Scientific World Journal, 8*, 873–882.

Parsay, S., Mosavi-Jarrahi, A., Arabgol, F., & Kiomarcy, A. (2011). Intellectual and behavioral impairment after chemotherapy and radiotherapy among children with cancer in Iran. *Asian Pacific Journal of Cancer Prevention, 12*, 1329–1332.

Ptácek, R., Kuzelová, H., & Stefano, G.B. (2011). Dopamine D4 receptor gene DRD4 and its association with psychiatric disorders. *Medical Science Monitor, 17*, RA215–RA220.

Rasmussen, P., Gillberg, C., Waldenström, E., & Svenson, B. (1983). Perceptual, motor and attentional deficits in seven-year-old children: neurological and neurodevelopmental aspects. *Developmental Medicine and Child Neurology, 25,* 315–333.

Richards, L.M. (2013). It is time for a more integrated bio-psycho-social approach to ADHD. *Clinical Child Psychology and Psychiatry, 18,* 483–503.

Rodriguez, A., & Waldenström, U. (2008). Fetal origins of child non-right-handedness and mental health. *Journal of Child Psychology and Psychiatry, 49,* 967–976.

Rosenhall, U., Nordin, V., Brantberg, K., & Gillberg, C. (2003). Autism and auditory brain stem responses. *Ear and Hearing, 24,* 206–214.

Rucklidge, J.J., Harrison, R., & Johnstone, J. (2011). Can micronutrients improve neurocognitive functioning in adults with ADHD and severe mood dysregulation? A pilot study. *Journal of Alternative and Complementary Medicine, 17,* 1125–1131.

Rutter, M. (1982). Syndromes attributed to "minimal brain dysfunction" in childhood. *American Journal of Psychiatry, 139,* 21–33.

Scott, M.N., Taylor, H.G., Fristad, M.A., Klein, N., Espy, K.A., Minich, N., et al. (2012). Behavior disorders in extremely preterm/extremely low birth weight children in kindergarten. *Journal of Developmental and Behavioral Pediatrics, 33,* 202–213.

Smits, M., Dippel, D.W., Houston, G.C., Wielopolski, P.A., Koudstaal, P.J., Hunink, M.G., et al. (2009). Postconcussion syndrome after minor head injury: brain activation of working memory and attention. *Human Brain Mapping, 30,* 2789–2803.

Spencer, T.J., Biederman, J., & Mick, E. (2007). Attention-deficit/hyperactivity disorder: diagnosis, lifespan, comorbidities, and neurobiology. *Journal of Pediatric Psychology, 32,* 631–642.

Söderlund, G., Sikström, S., & Smart, A. (2007). Listen to the noise: noise is beneficial for cognitive performance in ADHD. *Journal of Child Psychology and Psychiatry, 48,* 840–847.

Thapar, A., Cooper, M., Jefferies, R., & Stergiakouli, E. (2012). What causes attention deficit hyperactivity disorder? *Archives of Disease in Childhood, 97,* 260–265.

Weihe, P., Debes, F., White, R.F., Sørensen, N., Budtz-Jørgensen, E., Keiding, N., et al. (2003). [Environmental epidemiology research leads to a decrease of the exposure limit for mercury]. *Ugeskrift for laeger, 165,* 107–111.

Wester, K., Irvine, D.R., & Hugdahl, K. (2001). Auditory laterality and attentional deficits after thalamic haemorrhage. *Journal of Neurology, 248,* 676–683.

Wilens, T.E., & Spencer, T.J. (2010). Understanding attention-deficit/hyperactivity disorder from childhood to adulthood. *Postgraduate Medicine, 122,* 97–109.

Woodward, L., Taylor, E., & Dowdney, L. (1998). The parenting and family functioning of children with hyperactivity. *Journal of Child Psychology and Psychiatry, 39,* 161–169.

What Is the Outcome—Can You Outgrow It?

The prognosis in cases of ADHD and DAMP—and in most of the other disorders in the ESSENCE group—varies greatly (Barkley et al., 2006; Biederman, Petty, et al., 2012; Rasmussen & Gillberg, 2000). Some children do just fine as they grow up, and life can turn out very well for them. For others, the case is rather the opposite; life is filled with adversity and the only path that comes naturally is that of substance abuse, depression, anxiety, academic failure, unemployment, and crime. Naturally there are also many who have a prognosis somewhere in between these two extremes (Hodgkins et al., 2011).

THOSE WITH A FAVORABLE PROGNOSIS

What "favorable prognosis" means depends on what one refers to when using the expression. Whether one can function in society is one measure of prognosis, but it is not apparent how one defines the term "function." What the terms "functioning poorly" or "not functioning" refer to is more obvious. By analyzing what one means by "not functioning well in society" one can get, if indirectly, an idea of what it means to function well.

Many studies define "poor psychosocial prognosis" (basically synony-mous with not functioning well in society) as one or more of the follow-ing: criminal activity, substance abuse, mental illness, welfare dependency, lack of friends, long-term sick leave, and inability to provide for oneself. Some of these categories are, among other things depending on what soci-ety and time one is in, to be considered as more serious. In that sense, criminal activity is generally considered very negative, whereas the impli-cations of inability to provide for oneself naturally depend on factors such as the proportion of unemployed people in the society in question.

For those who do well (i.e., the ones who are well functioning in psycho-social contexts), none of the things associated with poor prognosis apply. Judging from this, it is probable that things turn out well for slightly less than half of everyone who during childhood has had problems associable with a DAMP diagnosis, and for slightly more than half of those who have been given the childhood diagnosis "ADHD" regardless of whether there have been problems with motor control present or not.

That "things turn out well" naturally does not mean that one is com-pletely free of problems. The majority of everyone with DAMP and many of those who have had "pure" ADHD have a lingering feeling that "some-thing is wrong," regardless of whether they were given a diagnosis during childhood or not. Deep down, many have, as has been mentioned several times before in this book, low self-esteem. This is generally a more specific low self-esteem than the one most of us profess to have in certain con-texts. Low self-esteem when it comes to ADHD/DAMP is often synony-mous with "feeling stupid" and manifests for example through refusal to do things, saying that one is unable or does not want to, and pulling away. One does not believe one has the energy to read books ("I probably can't read quickly enough and understand well enough"), go to the cinema or theater ("What if I won't manage to concentrate or read the subtitles?"), or take part in various physical activities ("I probably won't be able to catch the ball"). Some of these apprehensions may be well founded, but most of them concern functions that are no longer abnormal in the same way as they were during childhood. Many people with ADHD/DAMP never find out whether their original difficulties have subsided or disappeared completely. The fear of failing again, and above all the concern that one will make a fool of oneself in public, are too powerful.

Some people with ADHD have tremendously good self-esteem. Some have been that way for as long as they can remember; others have "fought their way there." There is no discernible common denominator uniting all of those with strong self-esteem. It might possibly be more common in the group with hyperactivity and impulsiveness than in the normal to hypoactive group.

The majority of people with ADHD/DAMP, even within the group that does not have a particularly good prognosis, live at least parts of their adult life in romantic relationships, and most of them form families and have children of their own. How things turn out for the children varies greatly and depends partly on whether the parent's problems are hereditary or not, partly on how well the parent has managed to adapt, and not least on how well the parent understands his or her own problems and thereby ideally the child's as well, if the child also has ADHD/DAMP.

THE MANY WITH A LESS FAVORABLE PROGNOSIS

From what has been said in the section on those with a relatively good prognosis, it is apparent that approximately half of everyone with ADHD functions worse psychosocially during adulthood and that any one of the signs of a poor prognosis previously mentioned is present.

Follow-up studies of children with ADHD/DAMP have hitherto not taken the term "quality of life" into adequate consideration. Not functioning perfectly psychosocially does not mean that one does not have a good life.

The rise of the computerized society, with high demands for verbal ability, good coordination, skill at multitasking, and speed, has probably meant that many people with ADHD/DAMP, who could earlier have been said to have a "favorable prognosis," must now be considered to have a "less favorable prognosis."

The vast majority of all individuals meeting the criteria for an early childhood diagnosis of ADHD will have some remaining inattention, activity control, or impulsivity problems throughout life. It is not true that many people with ADHD "grow completely out of it." Instead, there is a remaining feeling of restlessness, nervousness, and being high-strung and inefficient in many cases. The lack of good planning ability and difficulty keeping to time characterize a majority of all with childhood ADHD once they reach adult life. Even though only perhaps half of all with childhood-diagnosed ADHD still meet the full DSM criteria for the disorder in adult life, the vast majority still have some of the symptoms of the disorder. Inattention, distractibility, and poor planning (plus an inner feeling of constant unrest) are present to some extent in almost everybody in adult life. This may also be coupled with a feeling of inability to control temper that may instead, in some cases, have led to an obsessive-compulsive way of trying to control everything in life.

There are probably at least two major (and one smaller) subgroups when it comes to "poor outcome" in ADHD. One of these consists of those with ADHD plus early-onset ODD symptoms, sometimes followed by conduct disorder and antisocial personality development. The other major subgroup is the one with ADHD plus DCD; these patients tend to have autistic-type behavior problems and academic failure from school start onward. There is also a smaller subgroup with elements of both of the two mentioned groups. The ADHD+ODD group is the one that accounts for most of the antisocial development in ADHD, whereas the ADHD+DCD group is more clearly and directly associated with academic failure from the start. Both groups share poor outcome in terms of unemployment and inability to support themselves as adults, but only the former is strongly associated with antisocial development.

THOSE WITH MAJOR PERSISTENT PROBLEMS

The majority of those with a less favorable prognosis have very pronounced persisting problems of various kinds. This is on the one hand a result of many of the primary ADHD/DAMP/ESSENCE symptoms still remaining, but on the other hand it is also due to mental and social adjustment gradually failing in several key aspects.

Criminality and Severe Antisocial Development

A smaller group, a total of probably around 10% of everyone with ADHD/ DAMP/ESSENCE, has been arrested for criminal acts two or more times before about the age of 20 to 25 years (e.g., Rasmussen & Gillberg, 2000). This criminal activity has often been a matter of petty theft or had a direct connection to substance abuse or impulsive outbursts of aggression. Only in a few cases is it a matter of serious violent crimes and behavior that can be classified as typical of so-called hoodlums. Conversely, however, the fact is that many hoodlums in society—a small group, but one with enormously negative effects for themselves and other people—have a background with severe ADHD, DAMP, or other ESSENCE problems. Young violent imprisoned male offenders have an extremely high risk of ADHD, upwards of 60% of all cases according to several studies (e.g., Billstedt et al., 2013).

It appears that ADHD with ODD and conduct disorder accounts for a very large proportion of all substance use-related and impulsive violent crime, but that ASD, which, by and large, if anything, may be inversely correlated with substance abuse and criminal activity in adult life (Hallerbäck et al., 2012; Hippler et al., 2010), is linked to the very rare but extremely important phenomenon of serial killing (Allely et al., 2012).

Severe Mental Illness, Psychiatric Disorder, and
Personality Disorder

Approximately another 10% to 30% of everyone with ADHD/DAMP and other ESSENCE develop a set of problems dominated by severe mental illness during adulthood (Rasmussen & Gillberg, 2000). This group comprises young people with psychoses of different kinds, perhaps particularly with a manic-depressive/bipolar disposition or—in exceptional cases—of a schizophrenic character. These numbers tell us that many with the diagnoses manic-depressive disorder and schizophrenia have underlying ADHD/DAMP or other ESSENCE problems (Lugnegård et al., 2012; Unenge Hallerbäck et al., 2012). Many more have other serious psychiatric (including substance abuse-related) problems and meet the criteria for severe generalized anxiety disorder, chronic dysphoria or recurrent depression, and personality disorders of different kinds.

Academic Underachievement, Unemployment, and Driver's License

Regardless of their psychiatric problems, the vast majority of individuals with ADHD/DAMP who have a less favorable prognosis have great difficulties in reading and writing, lack higher education, and find it hard keeping a job (Biederman, Fried, et al., 2011; Rasmussen & Gillberg, 2000). Many also end up in accidents of different kinds. Young men with ADHD/DAMP are especially often involved in car accidents (Barkley, 2004). This has important implications for teachers at driving schools, who need to know that a substantial proportion of their clientele will have major concentration and attention difficulties that may interfere with their driving skills and aspects of security in traffic. Sometimes there is a need to communicate between the individual's medical doctor and the driving school teacher, and authorities may have a say in whether or not they will issue a driver's license to a person with ADHD whose symptoms are not well taken care of (including with medication and/or non-medication).

CONCLUDING REMARKS

Some individuals with ADHD/DAMP/ESSENCE manage relatively well in their adult years, and a smaller number have really excellent outcomes, leading independent, successful lives. Around half of all with a childhood diagnosis or problem constellation compatible with the diagnosis, though, fare much worse. Persistence of severe ADHD, depression and anxiety, social maladjustment, criminal activity, substance abuse, mental illness, and "personality disorder" are not uncommon. Difficulties in reading and writing and academic underachievement relative to IQ are the norm rather than the exception. Unemployment and difficulties holding down a job are extremely common in this group. Accidents are overrepresented and may cause particular harm when men in the 18- to 25-year-old age range are involved in traffic accidents. There is evidence to suggest that simple efforts such as screening, diagnosis, information, advice, and (not least educational) support could improve the childhood and adolescent situation for many in the group with a less favorable prognosis. In some of these cases, such efforts, together with medication, could affect the adult prognosis in a very positive direction. Given that "the ADHDs" and their many comorbidities constitute a huge public health problem, every individual who can be derailed from the pathway to mental ill health, major accidents, criminality, unemployment, and social exclusion to one of a more favorable outcome counts.

REFERENCES

Allely, C.S., Doolin, O., Gillberg, C., Gillberg, I.C., Puckering, C, Smillie, M., et al. (2012). Can psychopathology at age 7 be predicted from clinical observation at one year? Evidence from the ALSPAC cohort. *Research in Developmental Disabilities, 33,* 2292–2300.

Barkley, R.A. (2004). Driving impairments in teens and adults with attention-deficit/ hyperactivity disorder. *Psychiatric Clinics of North America, 27,* 233–260.

Barkley, R.A., Fischer, M., Smallish, L., & Fletcher, K. (2006). Young adult outcome of hyperactive children: adaptive functioning in major life activities. *Journal of the American Academy of Child and Adolescent Psychiatry, 45,* 192–202.

Biederman, J., Fried, R., Petty, C.R., Wozniak, J., Doyle, A.E., Henin, A. et al. (2011). Cognitive development in adults with attention-deficit/hyperactivity disorder: a controlled study in medication-naive adults across the adult life cycle. *Journal of Clinical Psychiatry, 72,* 11–16.

Biederman, J., Petty, C.R., Woodworth, K.Y., Lomedico, A., Hyder, L.L., & Faraone, S.V. (2012). Adult outcome of attention-deficit/hyperactivity disorder: a controlled 16-year follow-up study. *Journal of Clinical Psychiatry, 73,* 941–950.

Billstedt, E., Wallinius, M., Anckarsäter, H., & Hofvander, B. (2013) ESSENCE disorders in violent offenders. In progress

Hallerbäck, M.U., Lugnegård, T., Gillberg, C. (2012). ADHD and nicotine use in schizophrenia and Asperger syndrome: a controlled study. *Journal of Attention Disorders,* (Epub ahead of print, April 12).

Hippler, K., Viding, E., Klicpera, C., & Happé, F. (2010). No increase in criminal convictions in Hans Asperger's original cohort. *Journal of Autism and Developmental Disorders, 40,* 774–780.

Hodgkins, P., Arnold, L.E., Shaw, M., Caci, H., Kahle, J., Woods, A.G., et al. (2011). A systematic review of global publication trends regarding long-term outcomes of ADHD. *Frontiers in Psychiatry*, *2*, 84.

Lugnegård, T., Hallerbäck, M.U., & Gillberg, C. (2012). Personality disorders and autism spectrum disorders: what are the connections? *Comprehensive Psychiatry*, *53*, 333–340.

Rasmussen, P., & Gillberg, C. (2000). Natural outcome of ADHD with developmental coordination disorder at age 22 years: a controlled, longitudinal, community-based study. *Journal of the American Academy of Child and Adolescent Psychiatry*, *39*, 1424–1431.

Unenge Hallerbäck, M., Lugnegård, T., & Gillberg, C. (2012). Is autism spectrum disorder common in schizophrenia? *Psychiatry Research*, *198*, 12–17.

Intervention: Psychoeducation, Self-Help, Supportive Measures, and Treatment

I n cases of ADHD/DAMP and other ESSENCE it is often reasonable to talk about intervention or habilitation rather than treatment. Referring to intervention as "treatment" can be misleading as this implies a potential cure. ADHD/DAMP and most other ESSENCE can usually not be "cured." Alleviation of suffering and significant reduction of disability, though, are more or less always within reach, once the diagnosis is actually given (Nydén et al., 2008).

THE UNIQUENESS OF ALL INDIVIDUALS REGARDLESS OF CATEGORY OF DIAGNOSIS

All children, adolescents, and adults with ADHD/DAMP and other ESSENCE are unique individuals. All interventions must therefore, naturally, be individualized. No child can be "treated" solely based on the knowledge that he or she has an ADHD/DAMP, DCD, ASD, SLD, IDD, or Tourette syndrome diagnosis. When designing an intervention program for ADHD, one must, apart from the diagnosis itself and what it entails for that individual person, also consider what kind of family and social network the person is a part of, how school is working out for him or her, what associated problems there are, and what the person's core personality/temperament is like.

INFORMATION—ENABLING SELF-HELP

In the diagnosis "ADHD" itself—or in any of the other ESSENCE group diagnoses—thoroughly interpreted and reviewed—there is actually already a lot about "treatment" and "empowerment to self-help." The idea of making the diagnosis—on the basis of a sound and comprehensive assessment involving medical, psychological, educational, parental (or spouse or equivalent), and affected individual's information/observation—is to bring about an improved quality of life by providing insight into the person's difficulties and a change in attitude on the basis that it is possible to live with disorders without them being a major psychosocial handicap (Valente & Kennedy, 2012).

Oral information provided in conjunction with visits to a doctor, psychologist, language therapist, education specialist, nurse, or occupational therapist is valuable. Written information, possibly conveyed through relatively short information folders or slightly longer pamphlets on ADHD/DAMP, is also meaningful. Appropriate literature should also be recommended. The Internet is an important source of information; not least because of this fact, is it important to have the "right" name for the difficulties one would like to know more about (Mao et al., 2011).

Appropriate special interest associations can be an important source of information as well as provide support in a long-term perspective. Many families wish to be "anonymous" and do not want to be a part of associations that they find to be intrusive or overly enthusiastic. As a doctor or psychologist, one has to respect this attitude. Special interest associations rarely reach more than 40% of a disability group, meaning that a majority of those affected are usually not part of or a member of any association.

However, it should be mentioned that it is difficult to replace the sense of community and mutual experience that families with similar difficulties can offer each other.

An excellent way of helping the whole family is to organize a "family week" or "family weekend" during which, for example, five to 10 families—parents, children with ADHD/DAMP/another "specific" diagnosis in the ESSENCE group, and their siblings—gather together and learn as much as possible about the diagnosis, while getting to know each other in the process. Training in how one can learn to handle the child's behavioral problems, "tips" (such as lowering one's voice instead of raising it, being "consistent" rather than "too flexible," being concrete rather than vague, generally using fewer rather than many words when explaining things), and exercises of different kinds can be provided and performed in conjunction with these family gatherings. Variations on the theme of family week/family weekend, such as evening lectures or family camps, can also be very positive for the family and help alleviate a lot of stress.

DIFFERENT KINDS OF FAMILY SUPPORT

Economic and psychological-educational supportive measures for families who have children with ADHD/DAMP and other ESSENCE can be quite important in the overall care of the child.

Some families who have children with ESSENCE need financial support. It is important to mention that economic supportive measures should not be based on diagnosis but instead the individual family's unique circumstances and needs. For instance, no one can *demand* a childcare allowance and refer only to an ADHD diagnosis; the degree of disability and the extent of required supportive measures are what matter. The availability of such support varies from one country to another and from one region to the next.

Families' need for psychological support is also significant. Economic support can constitute a positive psychological effort but can never replace personal conversations or human understanding.

Families sometimes also need support in the form of consultations with a pediatrician, general practitioner, psychologist, child psychiatrist, or adult psychiatrist. A select few families may need family therapy of the more traditional kind, but the therapists must then either have adequate knowledge of ADHD/DAMP and other disorders in the ESSENCE group to be able to put the child's and family's problems into such a perspective, or be aware that the child has ADHD/DAMP and that one does not necessarily have to interpret the family's interactions the same way one would have in a family without children with ESSENCE.

A particular form of family therapy is the so-called Marte Meo method, which, among other things, includes the process of discussing and then planning and testing alternative strategies for solving problems, based on videotaped sequences of the child's behaviors and those of the rest of the family or those of the teachers. Correctly implemented, this method can be valuable, at least for dealing with oppositional behaviors associated with ADHD (Axberg et al., 2006).

One must, however, be aware that all more extensive family-oriented therapies are relatively resource-intensive and thus costly. For as many as possible of all those affected to be able to get help, one must generally focus more on considerably less resource-demanding efforts (Hinojosa et al., 2012). It is also important to weigh the pros and cons as regards "blanket-type" parent/family training support schemes that may be rolled out for whole communities in attempts to remediate "parenting problems" or support positive parenting for the whole population, including those with ESSENCE. Such programs may be very costly and have major, some, little, or no, or even negative effects unless they are properly evaluated and supported before implementation takes place (Wilson et al., 2012).

PEDAGOGIC INTERVENTIONS AND EDUCATIONAL SUPPORT

Almost without exception, children with ADHD/DAMP need pedagogic/educational support of different kinds.

Many children with ADHD/DAMP find it hard to devote themselves to any part of the type of education normally found in large classrooms if no particular measures have been taken in any way. Conversely, one should note that tutoring in many cases has great potential to provide even the most disabled student with ADHD/DAMP with adequate skills. This is difficult to discuss openly in a time when it is assumed to be a given that all children not suffering from IDD do just fine in classes of 30 to 40 children.

The majority of children with ADHD/DAMP would actually need to receive half or more of their education individually or in small groups. Instructions in one's mother tongue, writing, foreign languages, and mathematics would need to be individualized to a large extent, and this is difficult to put into practice in a large classroom. For homework to be done with any kind of efficiency, plenty of individual support is required. All experience shows that it is usually unfortunate when only the other family members help the child with his or her homework.

Many children with ADHD/DAMP would stand to gain a lot if schools could offer placement in smaller groups of 6 to 12 children. In such a group one could easily include children with many different types of ESSENCE disabilities and disorders, ADHD, DAMP, dyslexia, dyscalculia, Asperger syndrome, borderline intelligence, and also certain highly intelligent children for whom the type of education found in large classes does not present enough of a challenge.

If an affected child is assigned to a large classroom, it is often important for him or her to be seated near the teacher, preferably right next to the teacher's desk. This prevents the child from being constantly distracted by what other students are doing, and the teacher has an easier time noticing dips in concentration, misunderstandings, and other difficulties if the child is "right under the teacher's nose."

Children with ADHD/DAMP often cannot concentrate for more than about a minute at a time during their early school years. By the time they reach upper secondary school, their attention span may have been extended to around 15 or 20 minutes. These short sessions of concentration demand a great deal of imagination on the teacher's part in figuring out how to adjust the assignments so the child can complete them.

Regularly scheduled breaks are very valuable for many children, adolescents, and adults with ADHD. Most of them cannot handle (not even at upper secondary level or university) classes or lectures of 40 to 80 minutes in length. In rare cases there are students with DAMP (particularly when coexisting with marked autistic traits) who find it so difficult to shift their concentration/attention that they can, conversely, be hard to stop when they've been working on the same assignment for 80 minutes.

It is often said that all children with ADHD should have few stimuli around them in their learning environment and that decorations and irrelevant details should be removed from the classroom. This is accurate for a fairly large group of children with ADHD, but for others, those kinds of factors are of little or no importance: they could be learning at their best in a room where music is pumping out of the speakers and the TV is on. This means that one cannot give any general advice regarding "the optimal educational setting" in cases of ADHD/DAMP, or really any of the named disorders within the group of ESSENCE, other than that one must use trial and error in every individual case and that a majority of children (and adults) work better in an environment fairly low on stimuli. Having said that, it is also to be noted that "white noise" can actually augment the cognitive performance of some people with ADHD (Söderlund et al., 2007), although in others, reducing auditory stimuli improves working memory functioning (Sörqvist, 2010).

About half of all children with ADHD have a very "sluggish tempo" (Barkley, 2013) but would be able to perform relatively well if this aspect of their functioning were taken into account in the educational setting (Lundervold et al., 2011).

Bringing in a personal assistant can sometimes be a temporary solution to the problems that arise in children with severe ADHD/DAMP. The assistant can work as a support for attention and concentration and can, provided he or she has the pedagogic qualifications, help with assignments in, for example, English or mathematics. Unfortunately, personal assistants are sometimes viewed as a more long-term solution for problems associated with ADHD/DAMP. One must remember that the greatest problem for many children with ADHD/DAMP in the long term is if they haven't been given an adequate education. One must primarily make sure that children with ADHD/DAMP can learn as much as possible in school in order to boost their confidence and thus improve their future outlook. At best, a personal assistant can provide help in reaching that goal; other times, the assistant is only a way to put the child in a large class, without any actual learning being achieved along the way.

MOTOR CONTROL TRAINING, MARTIAL ARTS, AND YOGA

Clinical experience and limited research data suggest that some children with ADHD benefit from motor control training. These are primarily children with severe DAMP (i.e., those with the combination of ADHD and DCD), who generally have relatively pronounced difficulties in motor control, problems with coordinating their movements, and generally reduced muscle strength. For many of these, motor control training can be very valuable (Henderson & Henderson, 2003; Smits-Engelsman et al., 2013).

Discussion sometimes centers on who would best manage the motor control training and how it should be organized. This can certainly be subject to variation depending on the child's individual situation, the school's options, local alternatives, and the family's situation. It is important when planning the motor control training to adjust its schedule so that it does not conflict with other relevant activities, does not take up too much of the child's time, and is performed in such a way that the child can perceive it as something positive. All training that is perceived as something negative every time runs the risk of resulting in a partial or total absence of positive effects.

It can sometimes be good to have a physiotherapist or an occupational therapist involved from an early stage. The physiotherapist can, better than most, assess the child's motor control in an objective manner, organize a training program, and make sure that it is actually put into practice, through direct instruction or through supervision and guidance. It is especially important for the children with ADHD/DAMP whose difficulties border on cerebral palsy or other neuromuscular disorders to be referred to a physical therapist.

Some children have such major problems with their hand motor skills and fine motor skills in general that a specialized occupational therapist needs to be consulted. The child might need help with specific training of his or her digital motor skills and might in addition need aids such as pencil aids and an adjusted desk or chair at school/home.

Occupational therapists and/or physical therapists can sometimes offer so-called sensory motor integration training. The object of this is coordinating all types of perception (visual, auditory, tactile, kinesthetic) within and for the motor activity (Werry et al., 1990). There are many different variants of, and names for, the training. Some are very well intended and others are better described as a racket. In terms of motor control and perception, sensory motor integration training can be both stimulating and effective for some of the most impaired children with severe ADHD/DAMP. However, for many individuals with ADHD/DAMP, such integration training probably has only a relatively small positive effect and would take a lot of time away from other activities, including from reading and writing practice, which may be much more important for the individual's general adaptive development.

Executive functioning—often impaired in ADHD—can be improved by various kinds of martial arts programs (karate, kendo, aikido, judo) (Diamond & Lee, 2011). There is very little, if any, systematic study on the effects of martial arts specifically in ADHD, but the link between ADHD and executive function deficits makes martial arts "therapy" an interesting possibility. In the experience of the author, many patients and their parents and other relatives have reported very positive increases in attentional skills in children (and in some adults) with ADHD involved in regular judo or karate activities. It is high time for systematic research in the field.

According to a Cochrane review of the effects of yoga for neuropsychiatric disorders, there is limited (grade B) evidence for acute beneficial effects in ADHD (Balasubramaniam et al., 2013). In this field, too, intensified research on short- and longer-term effects of yoga on ADHD and ADHD symptoms would be welcomed.

A physical therapy group—or a martial arts group for that matter—at school can be of value to certain children and adolescents. In such a group, one could have, for example, three to 10 children with ADHD/DAMP and similar difficulties, under the supervision of a competent physical education teacher, practice movements, train muscle strength and posture, and also participate in ball games, something that would feel impossible or at least awkward in a large group of peers without ADHD/DAMP.

Depending on the competence and personality of the physical education teacher, some children can benefit greatly from simply participating in the regular classes with no special arrangements other than the teacher knowing which disorders are present.

Even though it is often possible to organize motor control training for children and adolescents with ADHD/DAMP within the regular school curriculum, it should at the same time be noted that many children with ADHD/DAMP benefit most from being exempted from physical education entirely. This often becomes a controversial matter. Some studies have shown that around half of all children relieved of physical education have ADHD/DAMP problems, and that the cause has been that the child has been ridiculed or bullied on account of his or her clumsy, immature, or awkward motor control. Hypotonia, low muscle strength, and mild ataxic problems also often contribute to the child not *daring* to perform the required tasks in physical education class. Not least does this kind of fear lead to one being teased and called a "chicken." One may need to try and remedy these kinds of problems by talking to the teachers and possibly also to the students in the classroom (without necessarily mentioning who the child with the problem is, but talking in more general terms). However, clinical experience shows that it is often impossible to make these situations reverse and turn into something good once they have arisen in the first place. Being relieved of physical education can then be the only solution. A not entirely uncommon cause of school refusal—or of truancy—in children and adolescents with ADHD/DAMP is, in fact, dread of physical education class. Children who are excused from gym class must have other opportunities to exercise and to train endurance and strength in their spare time or during the same time slot as physical education class.

INDIVIDUAL TALKS

From their teens onward, many with ADHD/DAMP and other ESSENCE would benefit from individual talks with a person with a great deal of experience of ADHD/DAMP. In earlier childhood years, many find it difficult to concentrate on conversations, which they can sometimes perceive as irrelevant or even completely incomprehensible.

A prerequisite for the talks to be meaningful is thus that the therapist has comprehensive knowledge of ADHD, DCD, or DAMP. It is hard for someone who has not familiarized himself or herself with the fundamental problems to understand why the person with the condition is not feeling well or how one is supposed to help with the problems. It is certainly fine if the talks are focused on insight, but they must generally also include significant elements of conclusion, concretization, and even advice and support.

For many teenagers with ADHD/DAMP/ESSENCE, it is their mother or father, a teacher, physiotherapist or occupational therapist, school nurse, friend, or a friend's parent—or even a police officer—who ends up in the role of conversation partner. Their efforts can be of crucial importance. However, they are much better equipped to be a strong support if they possess relevant knowledge of the neurodevelopmental disorder. Information pamphlets and books about ADHD—or another named disorder within the group of ESSENCE—can be useful in these cases.

CAN MEDICATION HELP?

Stimulants (Primarily Methylphenidate)

It has been shown beyond doubt that certain medications—primarily those with a stimulant effect—have exceptionally positive effects on core symptoms in cases of ADHD, at least if one applies a short-term perspective (Biederman & Spencer, 2008). The studies documenting such effects go back to the 1930s, and there are now thousands of reports on the hyperactivity-reducing and attention-improving properties of stimulants

such as methylphenidate and D-amphetamine. Several more recent studies also indicate that there are potential gains even in a more long-term
perspective, both as regards the outcome of the disorder itself and in terms
of health economics more generally (Fredriksen et al., 2013; Gillberg et al.,
1997; MTA, 1999; Wu et al., 2012). In spite of this, the prescription of
stimulants for ADHD/DAMP in many countries is still limited in scope.
In the United States and Australia, the situation is different: there, in some
states, as many as 10% or more of all boys in their school years are treated
with methylphenidate, amphetamines, or similar substances with stimulant effects. In most industrialized countries the use of ADHD medication
is below this level. In the early 2000s the trend in the Scandinavian countries has changed, and the rate of children with ADHD who receive medication with a stimulant has increased dramatically, but not beyond 1% or
2% of the general population of schoolchildren (Bilenberg et al., 2012).

How can it be that stimulants help in cases of ADHD/DAMP? And how
can it be that the attitude regarding whether one should use such medication varies so much? Should one even give medication that could also be
used as "drugs" to children?

Stimulants have been used to treat hyperactivity in children for
almost 80 years now. Hundreds of studies have documented the positive effects: better-organized activity, better concentration, and improved
learning ability. Acting-out behavior is reduced and fine motor skills are
improved when people with ADHD are medicated with methylphenidate.
The child becomes calmer and more composed and "listens better." The
negative effects have been few and are reversible, which means that if a person is taken off the medication, the side effects disappear without causing
any permanent harm. Weight loss and reduced need for sleep are, however,
very common. These problems can generally be handled by adjusting the
amount of medication and times of dosage. They are also reversible if the
treatment is terminated. Almost 70% of all children with ADHD experience a marked improvement when treated with stimulants, at least in a
short-term perspective. Several controlled studies that stretch over a year
or more indicate that around half of a group of children with severe ADHD/
DAMP benefit from the medication in a longer perspective of that kind.

Stimulants increase the activity of the brain's dopaminergic and noradrenergic nerve circuits (del Campo et al., 2011) (see Chapter 10), which according to physiological studies increases the alertness in the central nervous system. With increased alertness comes improved concentration. Improved concentration in turn enables one to better control one's activity level and behavior in general. Learning ability increases as well. These are probably the most important mechanisms behind the positive effects of stimulants in cases of ADHD. These are incidentally in principle similar in children and adults without ADHD; however, they are not equally apparent since those people do not have the same room for improvement—they are already well equipped, so to speak. The most common side effects (sleeping disorder and weight loss) are caused by the alertness increasing so much that it can be difficult to settle down in the evenings, along with stimulants having an appetite-suppressing effect.

It is important to highlight that the doses administered are relatively very small compared to those one would take to "get high." When it comes to amphetamine it is generally a matter of daily doses of 5 to 40 milligrams between the ages 5 and 15. Ritalin˚ and Concerta˚ (methylphenidate) are often administered in daily doses of 10 to 60 milligrams in the same age group. Short-acting Ritalin˚ may be given two, three, or four times a day and Concerta˚ may be given once a day. Other long-lasting methylphenidate formulations are also available. They still go out of one's system quite quickly and by the next day there are usually no lingering clinical effects.

The risk of addiction has been discussed at length. If the indicated dosage is used and there is adequate monitoring that the medication is used in the prescribed manner, there is probably no major risk of dosage increase or narcotic addiction. Millions of children all over the world have been treated with stimulants for the indication of ADHD, or for hyperactivity/difficulties in concentration/attention disorder, and little, if anything, suggests that they run an increased risk of substance abuse during adulthood. It is, if anything, more probable that the children who have been treated are at *less* risk of future substance abuse. This could be a result of the medication "protecting" them from psychosocial alienation. Further research in this field is required, though, to be able to determine to what extent stimulant treatment of children and adolescents with ADHD/DAMP can prevent difficulties in social adjustment during adult years.

Given the positive effects and the relatively mild side effects, it is fair to ask why not all children with ADHD/DAMP are offered treatment with stimulants. In the United States it is virtually standard procedure that, if an ADHD diagnosis is given, the clinician informs the parents about the possibility of—and also offers—such treatment. To some extent one can argue that the ADHD diagnosis itself has emerged as a result of the need for a diagnostic term for the difficulties, hyperactivity and difficulties in concentration/attention, that one has concluded could be alleviated by stimulants. This is one of several reasons behind why the term ADHD has been approached with a relatively large degree of skepticism in, for example, Sweden. Since the ADHD diagnosis "requires" only behavioral problems and not problems in motor control and perception, there is the risk that all kinds of behavioral disorders are thought to be ADHD and that stimulants will be prescribed relatively casually. Such a development is negative for many reasons, even if medication in small doses is relatively harmless. If there are a lot of stimulants in circulation in a community— for example, in the medicine and bathroom cabinets of every twentieth family with children in their school years (which is actually the case in certain places in the United States)—there is an increased risk that it can end up in the wrong hands and that a drug problem occurs as a result. If stimulants are seen as "first aid" there is a major risk that other measures, such as thorough diagnosis, information, advice, support, and pedagogic help, will be somewhat neglected. The difficulty in distinguishing between immaturity, for example in many boys, and mild variants of ADHD/ DAMP could also be significant and lead to many children being need-lessly medicated. These kinds of difficulties also raise the issue of the risk of over diagnosing children's problems more generally and hence the risk of medicalizing everyday problems.

For these reasons, among others, the prescription of stimulants to children for the indication of ADHD is still quite restrictive in Sweden. The treatment is reserved for children with severe ADHD who cannot get satisfactory help through only pedagogic, physical therapy, and psy-chosocial support efforts. Treatment with stimulants should, however, be considered in all cases of ADHD/DAMP for which more or less drastic alterations of everyday life are considered, such as changing schools, being committed to rehabilitation centers, or change of family home. Treatment with stimulants should also always be considered if other measures (diagnosis, information, pedagogic, and psychological efforts) do not seem to result in their set objectives.

If the decision is made to use treatment with stimulants, this must be performed under very carefully controlled circumstances. Parents, children, and the nurse and treating doctor concerned must have a good cooperation for the medication to work. With long-lasting methylphenidate and atomoxetine (see below) the treatment is facilitated since the school does not need to become involved in administering the child's medication. Attempts to terminate the medication should be made once a year. The medication is often terminated right at the beginning of puberty, but there is nothing to stop it from continuing for longer if there is a clear need for it. Everyone involved must be well aware of the side effects. Considerable weight loss and reluctance to eat can in some cases be reasons to end the medication, as can severe sleeping disorders, hallucinations (very rare), and severe tics. Headache is quite common in the beginning but usually disappears soon after finding an adequate dose. Heart rate goes up a little bit, as does blood pressure; this may rarely lead to the need to terminate medication. All side effects appear to be reversible, apart from possibly a certain small impact on the person's future height (0 to 1 centimeters off their height as an adult) in patients who have been treated for a very long time (many years). This means that one is probably not taking *any* serious risk by letting the child *try* the medication. There is, however, a widespread view that tics and Tourette syndrome can be provoked by treatment with stimulants. The majority of authorities in the field agree that stimulants can lead to increased tics in people who already have Tourette syndrome or are prone to tics, but that they are very rarely, if ever, provoked in individuals who would not otherwise have had them at a later time, had them in the past, or have mild and previously undiagnosed tics concurrently. Some children seem more depressed and introverted when they are on stimulants, and one may need to consider whether the disadvantages of the treatment outweigh the advantages. There is also a common observation that some children with severe ADHD/DAMP who are treated with a stimulant appear to become more "autistic," "in their own world," or withdrawn. On detailed analysis it often emerges that these are children who had autistic symptoms even before the medication started, and what one is seeing is how "obviously autistic" their symptoms are when the more obvious symptom of extreme hyperactivity and inattention is reduced.

One of the greatest obstacles for treating children with stimulants is of a psychological nature. "Should one really give drugs—even 'narcotic' drugs—to children?" is a common way of putting it that reflects the nature of the problem. Any medication that has come to be so strongly associated with drug addiction has a bad ring to it. It is not easy to use—and personally have faith in—a medication that one feels one must always "hide," explain, defend, or be ashamed of. Medication with stimulants cannot be carried out in a good way if not everyone involved (the parents, child, and doctor) agrees about the need for it and realizes that the reactions of those around one are something one has to expect.

Norepinephrine Reuptake Inhibitors (Atomoxetine)

Atomoxetine is a norepinephrine reuptake inhibitor (which among other things seems to selectively increase the function of dopamine in the frontal lobes); in large studies (short- and longer-term) of children and adults, it has been shown to be moderately to quite effective in controlling the symptoms of ADHD (Spencer et al., 2004). This medication has quickly become an important part of the treatment of ADHD, but it is still usually thought of as the second-line choice when it comes to medication. The side effects seem to be relatively mild—and partly similar to those with stimulants—and the substance is generally tolerated well. It has been suggested that suicidal ideation may be more common in individuals treated with atomoxetine than with placebo, but the evidence is difficult to interpret given that retrospective analysis of intent has clear limitations (Bangs et al., 2008).

In clinical practice, the beneficial effects of atomoxetine on core ADHD symptoms and overall behavior and functioning appear to emerge much more slowly than in the case of the stimulants. It may take weeks and even up to a month before the full benefits of atomoxetine medication can be properly assessed, much as with the use of some antidepressants for depressive disorder. In the author's experience, atomoxetine is not usually as well appreciated by the patients themselves as by their significant others (relatives, teachers, etc.). For adults, the rate of continued use of atomoxetine for ADHD over a longer period of time appears to be quite low compared to methylphenidate (Johnson et al., 2010).

Antiepileptic Medication

Antiepileptic medication can rarely be called for in cases of ADHD/DAMP, especially if there are symptoms present that occur in bursts or if the EEG shows epileptogenic changes (Schneebaum-Sender et al., 2012). One should start with a very low dosage and slowly increase it to avoid bothersome side effects. Beneficial effects may be long-lasting but more often than not are transient.

Some individuals with ADHD (sometimes with additional marked autistic features) have an EEG that meets or almost meets the full criteria for electric status epilepticus during slow sleep (ESES) (Larsson et al., 2012). They have bursts of continuous spike wave activity at night, and, even though this is rarely conclusively documented, they have reported episodes of odd movements and complete seeming paralysis in deep sleep. It is a matter of clinical controversy whether or not antiepileptic medication should be tried, but if other interventions and pharmacological treatments have not been effective, it is usually well advised to make a controlled trial over a period of about three months with an antiepileptic drug such as valproate.

Children with benign childhood epilepsy with rolandic spikes very often meet the criteria for ADHD (Tovia et al., 2011). In such cases, a trial of valproate or levetiracetam might well be indicated and successful in reducing ADHD symptoms as well as epileptogenic activity.

The subgroup of patients with ADHD with bipolar disorder should be considered for treatment with a mood stabilizer, with or without concomitant treatment with stimulants or atomoxetine. Lamotrigine and valproic acid should be titrated slowly with every-other-week (or more frequent) checkups by a doctor/nurse, either over the phone or in person.

Neuroleptics/Antipsychotics

Antipsychotics are medications that decrease the effect of dopamine in the brain. They are used occasionally in cases of ADHD but should generally not be considered if the child is not displaying any psychotic symptoms, extreme behavioral disorders, or severe tics. There are several side effects, and it is not uncommon for the ADHD/DAMP symptoms to deteriorate when using antipsychotic medication. In some cases, though, "new" antipsychotics (generally in small doses) can be very positive, even (in theory paradoxically) in children and adolescents who are being treated with stimulants.

Guanfacine and Venlafaxine

Both guanfacine (a noradrenergic agonist) and venlafaxine (a noradrenaline and serotonin reuptake inhibitor) have been used in the treatment of ADHD, and both have some preliminary support for efficacy. The evidence is perhaps less robust for guanfacine, and side effects may be more pronounced with this medication than with venlafaxine. Guanfacine is currently most used as a combination therapy drug, whereas venlafaxine can sometimes be effective when used as monotherapy for ADHD (Bukstein & Head, 2012; Ghanizadeh et al., 2013).

THE ROLE OF SLEEP AND TREATMENT FOR SLEEP DISORDERS IN ADHD

Stimulant treatments can be recommended perhaps particularly in the "primary" form of ADHD where there is usually some degree of hypoarousal and hypersomnia, whereas treatment of more primary forms of sleep disorders or of comorbidities (i.e., restless legs syndrome/ sleep-disordered breathing, bipolar disorders [with late-onset sleep], and epilepsy) might be the first choice of intervention if the hypoarousal state cannot be documented by history or in other ways.

Many individuals with ADHD (whether on medication or not) find it difficult to wind down at night, and they are usually not helped by advice such as, "Go to bed early and try to relax before you go to sleep." Physically exhausting activities are quite often helpful, and it may be a good idea to engage in exercise toward the end of the day.

Patients on stimulant medication may well be helped with their sleep problem by any of the following: (1) an extra small night-time dose, (2) a decrease of the afternoon dose, or (3) an increase of the 24-hour dose. If the stimulant is having good effects on daytime functioning, the usual way to improve the sleep cycle and settling down at night is *not* to decrease 24-hour dose.

Melatonin can sometimes be added to a stimulant to reduce total sleep latency and to increase the amount of sleep if adjusting the stimulant dose (either an extra small dose late in the day or decreasing the late afternoon/ night dose) has not led to good outcomes in terms of sleep (Mohammadi et al., 2012).

"ALTERNATIVE" TREATMENTS

Certain "alternative" medicines or supplementations are sometimes tested in cases of ADHD/DAMP. There is no conclusive documentation supporting their effectiveness. A small number of studies, some of which will not have been published upon the release of this book, indicate moderately positive effects of certain unsaturated fatty acids (such as omega-3) in people with ADHD/DAMP problems (e.g., Johnson et al., 2009; Richardson, 2012). Recent research—including some as yet unpublished studies of the effect of omega-3 on reading skills in the general population of children— suggests that young people with ADHD, who also have language and/or reading problems, might benefit considerably from supplementation with or an increase in food intake of fish oils.

The possible role of vitamin D has yet to be explored in proper studies. Vitamin D has been suggested to be a moderator of impairment in individuals genetically predisposed to ESSENCE (including ADHD), but there is no conclusive evidence at the time of going to press with this book.

In conclusion, one can say that the general view, at least outside of the United States, is that a considerable proportion of children with ADHD should not be treated with any medication. If medication is considered, there is no doubt that stimulants as stated above have a well-documented effect. Amphetamine and methylphenidate (sometimes the former helps, sometimes the latter) are the substances considered in this case. Other medications, specifically directed at the fundamental problems of ADHD, have little or no place in the treatment. However, children with ADHD can naturally sometimes need medications for entirely different reasons. It is important, then, to know that they—like all children with disorders in brain functions—are more likely to experience unexpected reactions. For example, the dosage may often need to be significantly higher or lower than what is indicated in the dosage instructions for children in general.

CONCLUDING REMARKS

A reasonable intervention program for *all* children with ADHD/DAMP—and for all children with any strong suspicion of any of the other disorders in the ESSENCE group—should include (1) screening of all the childhood-onset behavioral/psychiatric disorders included in the DSM or ICD diagnostic manuals, (2) diagnosis of the main/clinically most impairing conditions, (3) some further assessments of "comorbidities" (and "additional" diagnosis of them if relevant), (4) psychological testing/laboratory tests as indicated by the clinical diagnosis, (5) information about all the results of the comprehensive assessment taking into account the individuality of each patient, state-of-the-art advice (including about effects of diets, calorie intake, and exercise/physical training) to the patient, parents, and important others (including teachers), and (6) support (including educational) and follow-up as indicated in each individual case. Medication or supplementation (omega-3, vitamin D, etc.) may or may not need to be included as part of the intervention.

Interventions in ADHD and its associated problems in the domains of ESSENCE should target not only the disordered behaviors and neurobiology but also the strengths that are often present in some areas (e.g., "islets of special ability," "creativity," and certain memory skills, including the often intact or superior factual learning capacity). For example, behavioral therapies that depend on special skills, artistic or otherwise, and on superior memory skills in some areas could be enhanced by incorporating approaches that have been shown to improve learning and retention. Moreover, interventions should probably minimize the involvement of other functions that are compromised in the disorders (such as phonological processing and working memory, which are usually negatively affected).

Screening of ADHD/DAMP in conjunction with school start or during the first years of school of all children with learning or adjustment problems can be an important way of reaching children with ADHD/DAMP for whom the people around them have not yet reacted strongly enough for a diagnostic evaluation to have been arranged. An adjustment of the pedagogic situation at school is also virtually always necessary. Many children with ADHD/DAMP would need to be in smaller groups, although only rarely in "special classes." Teachers must be trained so that they are well versed in ADHD/DAMP problems. The question of motor control training is brought up in a significant minority of everyone with DAMP. Medication, usually for a long period of time, predominantly with stimulants, should be considered for an important subgroup—almost exclusively for those with severe ADHD/DAMP—with a marked degree of disability, and particularly when other interventions have not worked. One should not wait for a long period of time seeing problems increase and functions deteriorate without taking a stance on medication treatment.

One must apply a long-term perspective to the problems from the moment that the diagnosis is given. ADHD/DAMP rarely goes away completely, and for the majority it will be years before one can see signs of a more significant reduction of the degree of impairment.

REFERENCES

Axberg, U., Hansson, K., Broberg, A.G., & Wirtberg, I. (2006). The development of a systemic school-based intervention: Marte Meo and coordination meetings. *Family Process, 45*, 375–389.

Bangs, M. E., Tauscher-Wisniewski, S., Polzer, J., Zhang, S., Acharya, N., Desaiah, D., et al. (2008). Meta-analysis of suicide-related behavior events in patients treated with atomoxetine. *Journal of the American Academy of Child and Adolescent Psychiatry, 47*, 209–218.

Balasubramaniam, M., Telles, S., & Doraiswamy, P.M. (2013). Yoga on our minds: a systematic review of yoga for neuropsychiatric disorders. *Frontiers in Psychiatry, 25*, 117.

Barkley, R.A. (2013). Distinguishing sluggish cognitive tempo from ADHD in children and adolescents: executive functioning, impairment, and comorbidity. *Journal of Clinical Child and Adolescent Psychology, 42*(2), 161–173.

Biederman, J., & Spencer, T.J. (2008). Psychopharmacological interventions. *Child and Adolescent Psychiatric Clinics of North America, 17*, 439–458.

Bilenberg, N., Gillberg, C., Houmann, T., Kadesjö, B., Lensing, M.B., Plessen, K.J., et al. (2012). Prescription rates of ADHD medication in the Scandinavian countries and their national guidelines. *Nordic Journal of Psychiatry, 66*, 70–71.

Bukstein, O.G., & Head, J. (2012). Guanfacine ER for the treatment of adolescent attention-deficit/hyperactivity disorder. *Expert Opinion on Pharmacotherapy, 13*, 2207–2213.

Del Campo, N., Chamberlain, S.R., Sahakian, B.J., & Robbins, T.W. (2011). The roles of dopamine and noradrenaline in the pathophysiology and treatment of attention-deficit/hyperactivity disorder. *Biological Psychiatry, 69*, e145–e157.

Diamond, A., & Lee, K. (2011). Interventions shown to aid executive function development in children 4 to 12 years old. *Science, 333*, 959–964.

Fredriksen, M., Halmøy, A., Faraone, S.V., & Haavik, J. (2013). Long-term efficacy and safety of treatment with stimulants and atomoxetine in adult ADHD: A review of controlled and naturalistic studies. *European Neuropsychopharmacology, 23*(6), 508–527.

Ghanizadeh, A., Freeman, R.D., & Berk, M. (2013). Efficacy and adverse effects of venlafaxine in children and adolescents with ADHD: A systematic review of non-controlled and controlled trials. *Reviews on Recent Clinical Trials, 8*(1), 2–8.

Gillberg, C., Melander, H., von Knorring, A.L., Janols, L.O., Thernlund, G., Hagglöf, B., et al. (1997). Long-term stimulant treatment of children with attention-deficit hyperactivity disorder symptoms. A randomized, double-blind, placebo-controlled trial. *Archives of General Psychiatry, 54*, 857–864.

Henderson, S.E., & Henderson, L. (2003). Toward an understanding of developmental coordination disorder: terminological and diagnostic issues. *Neural Plasticity*, *10*, 1–13.

Hinojosa, M.S., Hinojosa, R., Fernandez-Baca, D., Knapp, C., & Thompson, L.A. (2012). Parental strain, parental health, and community characteristics among children with attention deficit-hyperactivity disorder. *Academic Pediatrics*, *12*, 502–508.

Johnson, M., Östlund, S., Fransson, G., Kadesjö, B., & Gillberg, C. (2009). Omega-3/omega-6 fatty acids for attention deficit hyperactivity disorder: a randomized placebo-controlled trial in children and adolescents. *Journal of Attention Disorders*, *12*, 394–401.

Johnson, M., Cederlund, M., Råstam, M., Areskoug, B., & Gillberg, C. (2010). Open-label trial of atomoxetine hydrochloride in adults with ADHD. *Journal of Attention Disorders*, *13*, 539–545.

Larsson, P.G., Bakke, K.A., Bjørnæs, H., Heminghyt, E., Rytter, E., Brager-Larsen, L., et al. (2012). The effect of levetiracetam on focal nocturnal epileptiform activity during sleep--a placebo-controlled double-blind cross-over study. *Epilepsy & Behavior*, *24*, 44–48.

Lundervold, A.J., Posserud, M.B., Ullebø, A.K., Sørensen, L., & Gillberg, C. (2011). Teacher reports of hypoactivity symptoms reflect slow cognitive processing speed in primary school children. *European Child & Adolescent Psychiatry*, *20*, 121–126.

Mao, A.R., Brams, M., Babcock, T., & Madhoo, M. (2011). A physician's guide to helping patients with ADHD find success in the workplace. *Postgraduate Medicine*, *123*, 60–70.

Mohammadi, M.R., Mostafavi, S.A., Keshavarz, S.A., Eshraghian, M.R., Hosseinzadeh, P., Hosseinzadeh-Attar, M.J., et al. (2012). Melatonin effects in methylphenidate treated children with attention deficit hyperactivity disorder: a randomized double blind clinical trial. *Iranian Journal of Psychiatry*, *7*, 87–92.

MTA. (1999). A 14-month randomized clinical trial of treatment strategies for attention-deficit/hyperactivity disorder. The MTA Cooperative Group. Multimodal Treatment Study of Children with ADHD. *Archives of General Psychiatry*, *56*, 1073–1086.

Nydén, A., Myrén, K.J., & Gillberg, C. (2008). Long-term psychosocial and health economy consequences of ADHD, autism, and reading-writing disorder: a prospective service evaluation project. *Journal of Attention Disorders*, *12*, 141–148.

Richardson, A.J. (2012). Review: ω-3 fatty acids produce a small improvement in ADHD symptoms in children compared with placebo. *Evidence-based Mental Health*, *15*, 46.

Schneebaum-Sender, N., Goldberg-Stern, H., Fattal-Valevski, A., & Kramer, U. (2012). Does a normalizing electroencephalogram in benign childhood epilepsy with centrotemporal spikes abort attention deficit hyperactivity disorder? *Pediatric Neurology*, *47*, 279–283.

Smits-Engelsman, B.C., Blank, R., vander Kaay, A.C., Mosterd-van der Meijs, R., Vlugt-van den Brand, E., Polatajko, H.J., et al. (2013). Efficacy of interventions to improve motor performance in children with developmental coordination disorder: a combined systematic review and meta-analysis. *Developmental Medicine and Child Neurology*, *55*(3), 229–237.

Spencer, T., Biederman, J., & Wilens, T. (2004). Nonstimulant treatment of adult attention-deficit/hyperactivity disorder. *Psychiatric Clinics of North America, 27,* 373–383,

Söderlund, G., Sikström, S., & Smart, A. (2007). Listen to the noise: noise is beneficial for cognitive performance in ADHD. *Journal of Child Psychology and Psychiatry, 48,* 840–847.

Sörqvist, P. (2010). The role of working memory capacity in auditory distraction: a review. *Noise & Health, 12,* 217–224.

Tovia, E., Goldberg-Stern, H., Ben Zeev, B, Heyman, E., Watemberg, N., Fattal-Valevski, A. et al. (2011). The prevalence of atypical presentations and comorbidities of benign childhood epilepsy with centrotemporal spikes. *Epilepsia, 52,* 1483–1488.

Valente, S., & Kennedy, B.L. (2012). Recognizing and treating adult ADHD. *Nurse Practitioner, 37,* 41–46.

Werry, J.S., Scaletti, R., & Mills, F. (1990). Sensory integration and teacher-judged learning problems: a controlled intervention trial. *Journal of Paediatrics and Child Health, 26,* 31–35.

Wilson, C., Thompson, L., McConnachie, A., & Wilson, P. (2012). Matching parenting support needs to service provision in a universal 13-month child health surveillance visit. *Child: Care, Health and Development, 38,* 665–674.

Wu, E.Q., Hodgkins, P., Ben-Hamadi, R., Setyawan, J., Xie, J., Sikirica, V., et al. (2012). Cost effectiveness of pharmacotherapies for attention-deficit hyperactivity disorder: a systematic literature review. *CNS Drugs, 26,* 581–600.

Who Can Help?

O ne of the greatest difficulties when it comes to ADHD/DAMP is that one cannot easily identify any single institution, doctor, psychologist, speech therapist, or teacher as primarily responsible for diagnosis and interventions of different kinds. To some extent, one can, of course, make the case that all illnesses and disorders are associated with similar difficulties, but the fact is that ADHD often comes with difficulties in so many areas that many different institutions *must* be involved in order for optimal help to be provided for the person affected. In these situations it is generally difficult to single out one organization and claim that it should have the chief responsibility and provide the coordination function.

Where they exist, institutions of school and school health care—in more general terms—should be coordinated and coordinating help efforts in the majority of cases of ADHD/DAMP and other ESSENCE. The condition is so common that it is unrealistic to imagine that a greater degree of specialization would be required in every single case. In young children with severe ADHD/DAMP problems, and many symptoms before the age of 6 years, well baby clinics and health visiting services would be the natural "first aid" institution.

SPECIAL INTEREST ASSOCIATIONS

The various special interest associations that can be considered in cases of ADHD/DAMP and other ESSENCE should be mentioned early in the interaction with individual families. Some families do not want to be involved with parent support groups or other interest groups targeting a specific diagnosis or group of diagnoses, but, for the majority, contact with a special interest group opens up a world of new information, opportunities to learn self-help skills, group meetings, conferences, and just "being part of the movement." Every clinician in contact with an individual or a family with ADHD/DAMP or other ESSENCE should make it part of his or her intervention program to provide brief oral—and written—information about appropriate support/interest groups. It is not the specialist's task to pressure a family to join a support group, but, currently, the value of considering specific support groups a part of the "treatment package" is often grossly underrated.

SCHOOL AND SCHOOL HEALTH CARE

It is most often in school that ADHD/DAMP and other ESSENCE problems get to be so difficult to deal with that some form of organized intervention program is considered necessary. School health care, when available, is therefore the natural institution to which children, family, and teachers should be able to turn and get help with an initial (usually preliminary) diagnostic assessment.

The school health care situation varies greatly within and across countries and regions, and it most likely does not function optimally anywhere with regard to ADHD/DAMP.

The ideal would be a situation where teachers or parents could turn to the school nurse when the question of ADHD/DAMP or other ESSENCE arises. The nurse could then see to contacting the school doctor and school psychologist, possibly also an education specialist with competence in the field of ADHD/dyslexia, and, if need be, other experts outside the school.

The school health care group, consisting of the nurse, doctor, psychologist, and education specialist, could also take care of screening for ADHD/DAMP (and dyslexia) during one of the first two years of school (at least among children presenting with an academic or behavioral/adjustment problem), so that children with mild to moderate ADHD/DAMP do not run the risk of going unrecognized.

The condition for school health care to be able to offer these help efforts is, of course, that there is adequate competence and enough resources to match the need. The school nurse has a central position since his or her role is perceived by most people as neutral. Doctors and psychologists with pediatric or "behavioral pediatric" training and special qualifications within the field of neuropsychiatry, neurodevelopment, and neuropsychology must be members of the school health team—and they must have sufficient time allotted to spend on these neurodevelopmental/ESSENCE problems—if it is going to be successful. Children and adolescents with ADHD/DAMP/ESSENCE (including language disorder and dyslexia) already use up a great deal of the limited resources of school health care as it is, but this does not always happen in a well-organized manner. An education specialist trained in the fields of ESSENCE must exist as a naturally integrated part of the school health care team. The education specialist is the team member best equipped to convey the results of examinations/diagnostic assessments and to make sure that supportive measures are taken within the school. This can primarily be done by drawing up an education intervention plan together with other teachers and with the student's parents.

There is much left to be done before school health care can function in this way. In many places, programs are being implemented in an effort to accelerate the development in the outlined direction. A collective educational effort would be necessary, as would central directives or advice that can clarify the important role that preschool/school health care can and should have in these respects. It is hard to imagine an alternative development in which more typical health care institutions (CAMHS, community pediatrics, behavioral pediatrics, child neuropsychiatry, and child habilitation) would assume the full responsibility of diagnostics, care, and follow-up of all children and adolescents with ADHD/

DAMP/ESSENCE, who, after all, represent several percent of the general population of children. The preschool and school with associated school health care have a natural role that should be used and not bungled or neglected.

CHILD NEUROPSYCHIATRY AND "GENERAL" CHILD PSYCHIATRY

Many parents of children with ADHD and other ESSENCE have been deeply disappointed by CAMHS or "child psychiatry" to which they have been referred; families have often felt that they have been criticized without receiving any actual help targeting the child's specific needs. One of the most important objections that parents have had is that the staff members at CAMHS assumed that the child's difficulties are a result of some kind of interaction problem within the family. These assumptions regarding causality have often been put forth without the child receiving a thorough examination. Unfortunately, there are still some CAMHS clinics where children with problems are not even examined by a doctor (or anyone else for that matter). This is, however, increasingly rare. It is now clear that a large proportion of the CAMHS clientele has ADHD/DAMP. The training and further education of CAMHS/child psychiatry employees is currently a high priority at many clinics throughout the world. One can hope that the awareness that some—indeed many—interaction problems can be the *result of the child's difficulties* and not the other way around will become more widespread in the near future. This should be the safest guarantee that, in the future, there will not have to be any basis for so many misunderstandings and feelings of guilt in the encounter between families and CAMHS within this field.

In "child neuropsychiatry clinics" (i.e., where the focus is on the presenting problems in the child), the assumption is generally that the child's problems and difficulties can bring about negative effects on the people around him or her. This has led to families turning to such units more and more for help with diagnosis, information, advice, and support. In a longer-term perspective these relatively limited teams of staff cannot be expected to take on the diagnosis and treatment of all children with ADHD/DAMP. The problem could be solved in at least two different ways. Either "regular" CAMHS/general child and adolescent psychiatry must generally be given so much information in the field of ESSENCE that cases of ADHD/DAMP can be handled there in a satisfactory manner, or one could instead imagine a major expansion of child neuropsychiatry departments and clinics ("ESSENCE teams," Fernell et al., 2012), closely linked to CAMHS but possibly with a more independent position.

CHILD HABILITATION

Within the field of child habilitation/behavioral pediatrics there are work models and a perspective of disorders and disabilities usually quite appropriate for children and adolescents with ADHD/DAMP and other ESSENCE. However, in some countries, habilitation services are now being separated from those clinics that take on the responsibility of diagnosis, and this can be a major problem. Diagnosis and intervention in the field of ADHD/DAMP and other ESSENCE should, preferably, take place in the same clinic.

ADULT PSYCHIATRY

The information about ADHD/DAMP and other ESSENCE is currently inadequate within the field of adult psychiatry (Nylander et al., 2013). A large portion of all child patients with ADHD/DAMP eventually become adult psychiatry patients. Many turn to psychiatry due to complications such as depression, anxiety, substance abuse, or social phobia. These latter conditions are generally appropriately diagnosed, but the previous history is not taken into account in a reasonable way and the ADHD/DAMP diagnosis is generally overlooked entirely (Nylander et al., 2009). It is still quite rare for adult psychiatrists to consider an ADHD/DAMP diagnosis or any of the other diagnoses within the ESSENCE group. This can be the case even if the patient was specifically treated under such diagnoses during his or her child and adolescent years. Adult psychiatrists should consider the possibility of ADHD in *all* patients with "personality disorders," substance abuse, psychosis, bipolar disorder, depression, or generalized anxiety disorder, and, indeed, in all cases deemed as complex and difficult to diagnose.

A comprehensive training program is needed to remedy this, what is perhaps the biggest shortcoming of the whole treatment/intervention field of ADHD/DAMP.

LABOR MARKET AUTHORITIES

Labor managing authorities and labor unions of different kinds often need to be involved in the habilitation of individuals with ADHD/DAMP. Currently one of the major problems is that employees within these institutions often have inadequate information about these disabilities. With improved knowledge within the labor market agency it would be easier to rehabilitate young—and sometimes certain older—people with ADHD/DAMP.

SOCIAL SERVICES AND CORRECTIONAL INSTITUTIONS

Within the local and federal institutions of social and correctional/detention services, and prisons, many children, adolescents, and adults with ADHD/DAMP are tended to without the diagnosis being known to the staff (Ginsberg & Lindefors, 2012). Sometimes the diagnosis has never been given, even though the set of symptoms is characteristic. In the future, a major effort needs to be made to spread knowledge about ADHD/DAMP and other neuropsychiatric problems in children, adolescents, and adults to people within these institutions in order to achieve optimal help efforts for the people treated there.

CONCLUDING REMARKS

Many social services and health organizations, from general social services, child and school health care, and child psychiatry/habilitation to correctional institutions (including prisons) and adult psychiatry, social services, and labor market institutions, need to be well informed in the field of ADHD/DAMP, and ESSENCE more generally, if help efforts for those affected are to be optimal. Preschool and school teachers need to be well versed in the normal development of children, ADHD/DAMP problems, and adequate education support measures if child care and school are not to contribute to further alienation of children and adolescents with ADHD/DAMP. Major educational efforts will be necessary over the coming years.

REFERENCES

Fernell, E., Landgren, M., & Gillberg, C. (2012). Organizational new thinking for children with cognitive disabilities. *Läkartidningen, 109*, 1555–1556.

Ginsberg, Y., & Lindefors, N. (2012). Methylphenidate treatment of adult male prison inmates with attention-deficit hyperactivity disorder: randomised double-blind placebo-controlled trial with open-label extension. *British Journal of Psychiatry, 200*, 68–73.

Nylander, L., Holmqvist, M., Gustafson, L., & Gillberg, C. (2009). ADHD in adult psychiatry. Minimum rates and clinical presentation in general psychiatry outpatients. *Nordic Journal of Psychiatry, 63*, 64–71.

Nylander L., Holmqvist M., Gustafson L., & Gillberg C. (2013). Attention-deficit/hyperactivity disorder (ADHD) and autism spectrum disorder (ASD) in adult psychiatry. A 20-year register study. *Nordic Journal Psychiatry, 67*, 344–350.

Case Histories of ADHD, DAMP, and Disorders in ESSENCE Group

ANDREW, 5 YEARS

Andrew's mother was convinced that there was nothing seriously wrong with her son's eyesight, even though he totally failed a vision test at the child health center. On his next visit the test went slightly better, and Andrew was unable to concentrate throughout the whole examination. The following was entered in his records: "Failed visual test. Concentration difficulties. Immature speech. No further concerns at follow-up." Andrew's mother felt relieved that the nurse did not suggest any additional investigation. This was in spite of her having long wondered whether her son was in need of help, on account of both his high activity and the difficulty getting him to listen.

That weekend Andrew went to stay with his maternal grandparents. For a long time his grandmother had sensed that "nothing" registered when she spoke to him. She felt that Andrew somehow did not listen, even though he looked her innocently in the eye and nodded when she admonished him. After he had pulled down and broken a glass decanter, she recounted the incident over the telephone to her daughter, who became upset.

On Andrew's return home his mother complained to him about his conduct while away. However, he did not appear to take any notice but merely fiddled with various objects absentmindedly. His mother felt that she had to grab hold of him to make him listen and even shake him to get his undivided attention. Nevertheless he continued to avoid her gaze. She felt desperate and shouted that she would go mad if he did not listen. Andrew's younger sister then began to cry. Meanwhile, he looked quizzically at his mother, almost as though he was seeing her for the very first time. His mother let go of him and began to cry herself. Andrew immediately announced in a hoarse, shrill voice that he was hungry, only to dash off to his room a few seconds later and start emptying all his toy boxes in a completely indiscriminate manner. His mother, who had just tidied up in there, ran into his room on hearing the sound of toys being strewn across the floor and was greeted by the sight of Andrew jumping up and down on a pile of clutter. She initially construed that he must derive enjoyment from this but, on seeing his vacant expression, realized that there was no pleasure to be had, only chaos.

Andrew's mother returned to the kitchen but, after a while, heard the sound of something breaking. When she went back into her son's room she noticed that a picture had fallen from the wall. Both the frame and glass were broken, and Andrew was bleeding from one of his fingers. Just as she was screaming that she had gone crazy and could not cope with this, Andrew's father came home and was surprised at all the commotion. She explained to him what had happened but felt that he was not listening. Andrew's father remarked that, as usual, she was exaggerating.

Comments

Andrew, in all probability, has ADHD or DAMP: he has attention deficits, concentration difficulties, and hyperactivity. His motor skills are most likely clumsy given what happens when he is alone in the room. His language and speech are immature according to the nurse at the child health center, and his voice is hoarse and shrill in a manner that is typical. He failed the vision test not because his vision is impaired, but because he is unable to concentrate.

The described problems are characteristic. It is also typical that no diagnosis has been made, despite Andrew's behavioral and linguistic abnormalities having been identified without difficulty at the child health center. Generally speaking, there is neither sufficient certainty in the medical assessment, nor any adequate training, which might have given the health center nurse enough professional self-confidence to raise the issue of ADHD/DAMP with Andrew's mother. For her part, Andrew's mother has long teetered between hope and despair and avoids bringing up problems if others do not flag them.

Further characteristic is the fact that Andrew's mother is the only one to comprehend that something is wrong. Andrew's father, who himself may have had ADHD as a boy and perhaps is still "immature," believes that Andrew's mother is simply being overprotective when wanting to discuss their son's problems. Andrew's grandmother has noticed that something is not quite right but has been unable to think of a good way of broaching the subject and does not know how to articulate her concern. Instead she gets irritated and directs her criticism toward her daughter, who feels that she is a rotten mother incapable of raising her children.

There is no question that a diagnosis would be enormously helpful in a case such as this one. Andrew's mother would have her fears confirmed—but also allayed. Her sense of guilt would abate and she would be able to channel her energy into understanding and helping her son instead of shouting and crying, or becoming swiftly dejected, as at present. Rather than denying all problems as he does currently, Andrew's father would need to revise his attitude and support her. Andrew's grandmother, who nevertheless is a huge support to her daughter, would get a chance to see her grandson's—and her daughter's—problems from an entirely different perspective and an opportunity to make sense of the diffuse anxiety that she herself has felt. All of this, however, would necessitate embracing a completely different attitude, both directly in relation to Andrew and among those closest to him. Andrew's problems would not vanish, but certain secondary complications (e.g., depression and conduct disorder) could possibly be prevented altogether.

For the family in question to have received optimal care, both the nurse and doctor at the child health center, or the pediatrician at the nearest children's outpatient clinic, would clearly have needed a sound knowledge of ADHD/DAMP and other disorders within the ESSENCE group. A child health center psychologist well versed in neuropsychology, together with the doctor and nurse, would have been able to enhance significantly the quality of help and support, which is undoubtedly called for in a case such as Andrew's.

BENJY, 8 YEARS

Benjy had failed to learn to read during his first year at junior school. He was capable of writing his name but would often write the letter "j" back to front. He was fairly quiet in class but could totally "flip" in the school playground; on such occasions he would simply rush round and round. Benjy appeared to be a dreamer, and unless one stood right next to him and said his name in a loud voice, it was practically impossible to catch his attention; both his mother and his teacher attested to this.

Benjy's parents had been particularly concerned about their son's development on two occasions: once when he was around 1 year old, and once in connection with a routine checkup at the child health center when he was 4. Benjy's mother remembered wondering, among other things, why he did not really look at her when she had tried to attract his attention at the age of 1. She had had his hearing tested but this was declared normal. During the checkup at the age of 4, Benjy's speech had been unclear and he had refused to draw a man (a standard developmental test). Throughout he had sat on his mother's lap sulking and sucking on his thumb. His mother felt that the health center nurse had been insensitive and had misunderstood Benjy. At the same time, though, she suspected that the nurse had been right about her son being slightly immature and having difficulty concentrating.

In more recent years, however, Benjy's parents had not worried. Benjy was the apple of his mother's eye and she felt a desire to shield him from all of the unpleasant things in life. It therefore came as something of a shock when, in the spring term of Year 4, his teacher intimated that he was in definite need of help. His mother became defensive and pointed out that Benjy seemed happy, went willingly to school, and had friends. Even so, his teacher was of the opinion that his reading, writing, and concentration difficulties were so great that remedial teaching needed to be implemented. She also wanted to discuss whether it was actually feasible for Benjy to receive the help that he required in his current class. Benjy's mother tried to keep her temper but became incensed when the teacher suggested that her son undergo testing by the school psychologist. She retorted that testing would not in fact be necessary, and that her son was certainly not some disturbed kid, which she felt was what the teacher was trying to imply. Benjy's mother walked away from the conversation with the situation unresolved, feeling as though her whole world had collapsed. She recalled someone once remarking that her brother, who had been unable to read or write at the age of 10, and who had been taught in a remedial class, was "mentally retarded" and now wondered whether this was what Benjy's teacher had been endeavoring to tell her—that Benjy had a learning disability. Things, however, had turned out well for her brother: he owned a car repair shop and had employees and could hardly be considered "thick."

A few days later the school nurse telephoned to say that she had made an appointment for Benjy and his mother with the school doctor in a week's time. By this stage, Benjy's mother had calmed down and felt that it would be helpful to have the opportunity to speak with someone impartial. Nevertheless, she was surprised when it transpired that a full hour had been scheduled for the appointment. Once the medical interview was over and Benjy had been examined, the doctor said that he believed that Benjy had ADHD with DCD (i.e., DAMP). When he described what the condition involved, Benjy's mother recognized nearly all of her son's symptoms: his concentration difficulties, his attention deficits, the fact that he never seemed to listen, his clumsy motor skills, and his reading and writing problems. Before leaving she was given a booklet on ADHD/DAMP to take home with her.

That evening Benjy's parents read the booklet and agreed that DAMP had to be what their son had. However, they could not understand why no one had said anything until now. In all likelihood this was not entirely true; it was more conceivable that no one previously had had a name for Benjy's problems. In retrospect, his mother felt—his father reported that he could not recall this as vividly—that Benjy had shown clear symptoms of DAMP when he was just 1 year old.

Several days later the school nurse rang Benjy's mother at work to seek her permission to arrange an assessment with the school psychologist. Benjy's mother was still averse to the idea but, since both the nurse and doctor appeared to know what they were talking about, gave her consent anyway. She stressed, however, that it would purely be a case of a single appointment, as she did not want Benjy made to think that he was "thick."

In the event, the visit to the psychologist went very well and Benjy's mother realized that she had harbored many preconceptions that were unfounded. A week later, when Benjy returned for a second appointment to complete the testing, he and his mother were given some information. They were told, among other things, that Benjy was of normal intelligence, something that his mother was relieved to learn. The test results also indicated that Benjy had dyslexia, and the psychologist wanted to meet with his teacher, the doctor, and the nurse to agree on the diagnosis and on a remedial program.

A further week later all parties attended a meeting. Both parents were present but on this occasion not Benjy. The doctor confirmed that Benjy's diagnosis was DAMP with concomitant dyslexia. Benjy's parents had read in their booklet that dyslexia was common in ADHD/DAMP. They were also told that ADHD/DAMP and dyslexia were common generally and that there is at least one child, sometimes two, with either condition in every classroom. Benjy's parents were relieved to hear this—it meant that their son was not that different, and his problems were not that bizarre.

It was agreed at the meeting that Benjy, accompanied by his mother or father, would visit the doctor a few days later to be given information about his diagnoses. In the meantime Benjy's teacher, together with a special needs teacher with dyslexia expertise, would develop a suitable educational intervention plan. Once the two of them had done this, they would discuss their recommendations with the school health team: the nurse, doctor, or psychologist—or all three.

Following the meeting Benjy's mother was glad that her son's teacher had not allowed herself to be deterred by her initial reaction. Within a matter of only a few weeks everyone had acquired a completely new picture: not of Benjy, but of his difficulties. Soon Benjy would obtain similar insight too.

Comments

Benjy has ADHD, DCD (i.e., DAMP), and dyslexia. Given that he does not have hyperactivity, it should come as no surprise that his difficulties had not been properly identified prior to the end of Year 4.

Benjy's comparatively late diagnosis is likely to be compensated for by the exemplary way in which his problems are now being addressed. It is evident that the staff at Benjy's school work in a well-thought-out manner and are sufficiently capable of diagnosing and catering for the type of difficulties he has. Moreover, the school health team (i.e., the nurse, doctor, and psychologist), in close collaboration with the teachers, appears to have enough time and staff to be able to devote to the problems in question. Ideally, school health services throughout the country should receive training and adequate resources to enable them to work in accordance with a similar model. However, for remedial work to be meaningful in cases such as Benjy's, there must be sufficient numbers of experienced special needs teachers in each local education authority.

CARL, 10 YEARS

Carl was the class clown. He would answer each and every question without bothering to raise his hand—he simply could not keep the answer to himself. When he answered, he was wrong as often as he was right. He had a habit of rocking on his chair and quite often rocked so violently that he would fall off in the middle of a lesson—frequently resulting in pandemonium. He would also chat incessantly to his classmates seated nearest him; when he was rebuked, it seemed not to have the slightest effect. At a parents' evening, one mother had insinuated that Carl was deliberately troublesome, although his teacher did not feel that there was anything "spiteful" about him.

Carl's mother and his teacher had had a number of run-ins with one another during his first two years at junior school. Initially, Carl's teacher had been certain that there must be something going on at home that was making him "unwell." Carl's mother consequently inquired what his teacher meant by "unwell"—she personally was convinced that Carl was exceptionally healthy. Unlike his elder brother and younger sister, both of whom had had many infections, he had never been ill. Carl's teacher replied that one could tell when a child was unwell by his or her behavior. She added that hyperactivity and rowdiness were symptoms of nervousness, worry, and anxiety, and said she was concerned that Carl was ridden with angst. His mother found this comment extraordinary since, in her opinion, Carl was both happy and affectionate. She did agree, however, that he was extremely active and that this could occasionally become wearing.

Carl's teacher had attended a series of talks on abused children. While attending these she had heard, among other things, that the very "symptoms" that Carl had should raise concerns about his welfare—perhaps he was not alright, perhaps he had been party to something that he needed to "act out." She had become particularly fixated on the idea that abuse of various kinds often gave rise to the *exact* problems she felt Carl had. However, even though she could see the "symptoms" that Carl displayed, she was unsure how to proceed since his mother denied all problems. She decided to approach the school psychologist, who recommended that Carl's mother contact child and adolescent mental health services. Carl's mother refused to do so as she was of the opinion that such services were intended for children with major problems, which she did not feel her son had.

Toward the end of the summer term of Year 4, it transpired that Carl had failed to learn to read at the same pace as his classmates. Carl's mother and his teacher subsequently fell out with one another to such a degree that a public row ensued, during which Carl's teacher became so agitated that she could not help but raise the issue of abuse. Although she did not consider it her place to mention this, the fact that Carl's mother appeared to be in such denial of her son's problems made her angry. Furthermore, her own concern for Carl had become so great that, during this row, she told his mother that his symptoms could indicate that he had been sexually abused. Carl's mother, who had not expected to hear such a remark, was rendered speechless and could only utter "Is that so?" before walking away without another word spoken.

The following day Carl's mother telephoned child and adolescent mental health services to make an appointment. When she explained precisely what had prompted her to ring, she was put through to a doctor in the outpatient clinic, who felt that she and her son should attend that very afternoon.

Two weeks later, immediately prior to school breaking up, a meeting was held that was attended by Carl's mother, Carl's teacher, and the doctor and psychologist from the child and adolescent mental health team. The doctor informed those present that Carl had ADHD. By this stage, Carl's mother had already encountered the term several times, but it was completely unfamiliar to Carl's teacher. The doctor went on to say that Carl's motor problems were possibly sufficiently pronounced to warrant a diagnosis of DCD. Carl's teacher had not heard of this term before either and felt that the conversation seemed mainly to revolve around a stupid acronym—in her view, Carl had a severe disorder. During the meeting the psychologist discussed the results of Carl's IQ test: he was of normal intelligence, albeit with an uneven cognitive profile; he also had concentration difficulties as well as certain perceptual problems. Carl's teacher felt that this tallied with her own observations but was astounded that the doctor and the psychologist were firm in their opinion that Carl had not been subjected to any serious abuse, sexual or otherwise. Carl's teacher was given a booklet on ADHD/DAMP to take with her from the meeting, and it was decided that they should all reconvene at the start of the autumn term.

Throughout the summer both Carl's teacher and his mother, independently of one another, read all the literature on ADHD, DCD, and DAMP that they could lay their hands on. It became apparent to Carl's teacher that Carl did indeed have ADHD with DCD (i.e., DAMP). Aside from his hyperactive behavior, she had also noticed that his motor skills and perception were immature. As for Carl's mother, it was harder to accept that her son's problems were something that could be regarded as abnormal.

However, when she read in a booklet that "normal" boys could be late maturing and have many of the behaviors that characterize those diagnosed with DAMP, she grew more positive toward her son's diagnosis. Moreover, she felt that a diagnosis of DAMP better encapsulated his problems than a diagnosis of ADHD.

On the first day of the autumn term, Carl's teacher spoke with his mother and apologized for having blurted out her suspicions during the row they had had the previous term. Carl's mother felt that she was now in a better position to understand, and that it was not quite so strange for her son's teacher to have been concerned the way she had been. Following this conversation Carl's mother and his teacher were able to start working together.

Carl's problems did not diminish, however, and he became more hyperactive during Year 5. This was in spite of him now having a diagnosis, and in spite of his parents and his school being able to address his difficulties and behavior in a more sympathetic and considered manner. Stimulant medication was discussed, but Carl's mother was reluctant at first. Her son's problems continued during Year 6 and, consequently, treatment with stimulant medication was commenced, which resulted in his hyperactivity decreasing dramatically.

Comments

The case of Carl illustrates a common problem; namely, that neuropsychiatric problems in children are assumed to be due to adverse social and psychological circumstances. Sexual abuse is a frequent "misdiagnosis" in ADHD/DAMP.

At the same time it should be said that it is neither strange nor wrong for the suspicion to arise, since social and psychological problems may very well give rise to symptoms that are *relatively* similar to those encountered in ADHD/DAMP. Furthermore, it goes without saying that it is possible for children with such diagnoses to be subjected to abuse of various kinds; ADHD/DAMP does not render them immune. Indeed, it is highly probable that children with these diagnoses are more at risk than other children.

Nevertheless, provided that the child himself or herself does not dis-
close any information or indicate in some other way that one might be
dealing with a case of abuse, it is important always to heed the following: symptoms such as hyperactivity, concentration difficulties, and attention deficits should not be primarily suspected of being connected with
abuse situations of various kinds.

The case also illustrates the disproportionate emphasis placed on psychosocial causal factors during initial and advanced teacher training. It
is a cause for regret that teacher training does not include fundamental
information about normal—and abnormal—child development. ADHD
and DAMP are problems that affect at least one child in every classroom.
In spite of this, the majority of all teachers lack the faintest idea of what
these diagnoses involve. Conversely, nearly all teachers have heard that
sexual abuse can give rise to symptoms such as hyperactivity, concentration difficulties, and lack of impulse control. One of the most common
causes of such symptoms is ADHD/DAMP; only in exceptional cases will
sexual and other kinds of abuse be the primary cause of such symptoms.

Learning about child and adolescent development, as well as about developmental abnormalities, should naturally form a significant part of teacher
training. It is unacceptable in the future for teachers to continue to remain the
only category of child experts in society not to be educated about children.

The case of Carl also demonstrates that correct information can bridge
many difficulties. It was only when both Carl's mother and his teacher
possessed similar knowledge that they were able to communicate and
start working as a team. Finally, while communication on equal terms
between parents and teachers is vital if child-oriented interventions are to
be meaningful, it is clear that this does not signify that all problems will
vanish simply because such dialogue has been established.

DANIEL, 15 YEARS

Daniel was depressed and too tired to go outside, too tired even to leave
his own room. Moreover, he could barely muster the energy to respond to

his parents' and siblings' questions, and did not believe he was capable of finding words to describe everything that felt wrong. A year earlier he had pilfered 40 oxazepam (a prescription drug for anxiety) tablets from his maternal grandmother's bathroom cabinet. In a letter that he had left on his father's desk—in the hope that someone would find it before it was too late—he had written that he wanted to "sleep for a long time."

Daniel felt silly when, accompanied by his mother, he went for an appointment at the child and adolescent psychiatry outpatient clinic. He disliked the fact that his mother spoke about his problems but, since he himself would never have been as forthcoming with the doctor, felt that it was good nonetheless that as much information as possible was disclosed. He became aware that his mother had not realized he had been depressed for a very long time and that, for several years, he had felt stupid and worthless. For a long while—and not solely on the occasion when he had helped himself to the tablets, or in the months prior to the appointment— he had contemplated whether life was actually worth living, but had not let on to others that he had given up.

During the consultation Daniel's mother recounted a number of things that her son could not recall. Daniel learned that he walked at an early age, at just nine months, and that he was constantly running around, unable to sit still. His mother also reported that he somehow never listened and that he did not speak an awful lot before the age of 3, although he subsequently made up for this. However, his speech had been unintelligible to everyone bar his immediate family and, between the ages of 4 and 6, he had seen a speech therapist. Daniel's mother was also aware that his father's childhood speech had been unclear—and delayed. Daniel wondered whether this might have any connection with his own problems.

The doctor asked whether Daniel had difficulty "finding words" and remembering names. Daniel was astonished that she could know this— this was something he found hopelessly difficult. Sometimes he would have all the words in his head, and could practically *see* them flying by, but was unable to catch hold of them at the precise moment they were needed. He also realized that he did actually know the names of many people, or cities in the case of geography, but just when someone asked he was incapable of uttering the answer.

Daniel's mother additionally stated that her son had always appeared intelligent, despite him having experienced major problems with both concentration and unclear speech. At school his teacher initially seemed to share this belief, but later—when it transpired that Daniel had difficulty spelling and writing neatly—it was as though she had tired of him. Daniel had loved his first year at junior school but subsequently felt that it had become increasingly boring. By the time he was 8 years old he was able to speak clearly but would stammer slightly when he became eager. At that age he could also read reasonably well—as well as his classmates—but found spelling incredibly hard.

Daniel had always hated PE. He also disliked skiing, skating, and playing ball games. At times his mother had wondered whether he was a little clumsy but had not known what was normal for boys his age. Besides which, he had appeared to be fairly dexterous on the rare occasions that he could concentrate on the things he liked, such as building electrical circuits and doing jigsaw puzzles.

Daniel had not had a single friend since he was 10 years old. Prior to this there had been boys his age who liked him and let him "hang out" with them. From the age of 11, however, Daniel had grown increasingly quiet and somehow "distant." He had mostly wanted to stay in his room, where he would often stand at the window watching children playing in the street. To family members he had appeared untroubled, although he was perhaps slightly more irritable than he had been previously. His family had not considered this a significant problem, although Daniel personally felt that this had been a dreadful period; he had not wished to become irritated but had been unable to prevent himself from snapping at his parents and siblings.

At school things had gone from bad to worse for Daniel. His mother found this odd given that he read so much, books as well as comics. Furthermore, he always kept books at his bedside, both fiction and non-fiction. Daniel enjoyed reading but felt that what he read did not sink in as well as he would have liked.

Once his mother had finished speaking, she was asked to leave the room and the doctor talked to Daniel in private. The doctor also carried out some tests. Among other things, Daniel had to hop on one leg and wave his hands around. He thought that the tests were strange and found it embarrassing that he had been obliged to get undressed. A few days later he underwent testing conducted by a psychologist. He actually found this quite enjoyable and, on departing, felt better than he had done in a long while.

A further week later Daniel and his mother returned to see the doctor and the psychologist. The doctor explained that Daniel had DAMP and dysgraphia, and possibly also dyslexia. In addition, he was suffering from depression. The psychologist stated that Daniel was highly intelligent and that his IQ score bordered on the range termed "very superior intelligence."

The investigation, diagnosis, and ensuing information resulted in Daniel starting to feel better. After two months, however, the doctor judged that he was still depressed and antidepressant medication was therefore commenced. At the same time the doctor and the psychologist did their best to inform Daniel's school about his difficulties. At a follow-up appointment six months later, Daniel felt pretty good and had even begun to seek the company of his classmates—something he had not envisaged—who accepted him within their group and did not tease him. In view of how long he had been depressed, the doctor thought that Daniel should remain on his medication for another few months before it was discontinued. Throughout the year following his diagnosis, the doctor had several individual chats with Daniel.

The family relinquished contact with child and adolescent mental health services after just over a year. When the doctor telephoned two years later, shortly after Daniel had turned 18, both he and his mother reported that "everything" was "quite OK."

Comments

The basis for the development of Daniel's depression lay in the fact that his DAMP problems had remained undiagnosed for many years. To his own and others' amazement, he turned out to be extremely intelligent. His IQ, which was around 127, would have been even higher had he not scored so poorly on the "Coding" and "Digit Span" subtests, which is very common in patients with ADHD and DAMP. Somehow everyone had suspected that Daniel had potential but, even so, he had been perceived as a failure at school—a belief that he in particular held.

EMMA, 16 YEARS

Emma had always had difficulty mixing with her peers. She would want to do everything her way, not deviating from her routines. Even when she was very young she had stood out as stubborn, inflexible, and somehow negative. Her parents worshipped her in spite of the fact that she was often cross, sullen, and even angry. Furthermore, she would frequently refuse to cooperate when anyone made demands on her. To the outside world she would initially come across as an unremarkable and impersonal individual, yet within her own family she was, if anything, domineering.

Emma had been late learning to talk properly and her voice had been conspicuously hoarse and monotonous from the outset. During a routine checkup at the child health center when she was 4 years old, she had refused to draw. Consequently, Emma's mother had been unsure whether her daughter was capable of drawing a man. Emma also refused to make eye contact and would sometimes shield her eyes with her hands if anyone outside her family tried to catch her gaze. For a while in Year 3 she had completely refused to talk to anyone other than her mother. During this time the only way that she could be persuaded to break her silence was by doing something new or particularly enjoyable with her; in such instances, it was as though she had forgotten all about her resolve not to speak. Her near-total muteness had gradually petered out but, outside her family and her immediate circle of friends, Emma had always been perceived as shy, reserved, or "moody." She had a couple of friends whom she had known since she was 2, with whom she spoke a great deal.

Throughout her first years at primary school, Emma had experienced major difficulties learning to read and write. It was as though she would be sitting thinking of something else and feel that she had been interrupted when asked a question by her teacher. When she was asked something, she would practically flinch and shoot her teacher an almost reproachful glare.

It was only when Emma was on the verge of leaving secondary school that everyone, including her mother and her form teacher, realized that something had to be done to help her. It was clear that she was scarcely capable of going on to study at sixth-form college, and so the school doctor referred her to a child neuropsychiatry clinic.

Following assessment on an outpatient basis over a period of one month, a total of five appointments, Emma was diagnosed with severe DAMP and selective mutism in partial remission. She had an IQ of 72 and, moreover, a very uneven cognitive profile; her verbal intelligence fell within the range of mental retardation. After much discussion, Emma was able to commence at a vocational special school just a few days after her 16th birthday. Six months later she was doing relatively well there and was one of the ablest in her group.

Emma's DAMP diagnosis came as an enormous relief to her mother and her form teacher, both of whom had been greatly concerned over the years without ever realizing that Emma had a genuine disability. Nevertheless, both suffered from a sense of guilt and wondered whether Emma might have fared even better in life had her difficulties been identified earlier.

Comments

Emma's case illustrates the common plight of many girls with DAMP; namely, that their fundamental difficulties are not detected whatsoever. According to a note in her school health records, a locum school doctor had considered a diagnosis of selective mutism when Emma was 10 years old. However, no one had picked up on the fact that she had DAMP, borderline intelligence, and an uneven cognitive profile.

There is no question that Emma's difficulties were sufficiently severe for her to have benefited immensely from being taught in a small group, or from attending a special school, from as early as primary school age. Instead she had always been placed in large classes. She definitely does not have "formal" mental retardation—her overall IQ is above 70 (see Chapter 2)—but her level of functioning is such that placement in a special school is by far the best option. Emma's shyness, reserve, and residual symptoms of selective mutism had completely vanished after she had been at her new school a year.

FREDDIE, 26 YEARS

Following his time at sixth-form college, which Freddie had often found hellish, things had improved for him. He worked for some years at a hamburger restaurant before resuming his studies. The reading and writing difficulties that he had always had persisted, but the mix of practical and theoretical elements made life a little easier. Furthermore, his course tutor had shown understanding and had promised early on that, should Freddie need an extra term or two to complete his nursing training, this would not be impossible to arrange. Consequently, Freddie had been able to relax to the extent that his studies were at least not rendered any more difficult by the stress and near-constant anxiety he had suffered from in secondary school and at sixth-form college.

Freddie went to see his GP to find out whether there was any medication that might help him sustain concentration while studying. He also wanted to discuss alcohol—he had noticed that drinking made it easier for him to talk to other people in a group, but also made him clumsy and made him slur his speech. Freddie's girlfriend wondered why he could not "hold his drink," although he personally did not consider himself unable to tolerate alcohol. He realized, nonetheless, that alcohol—in various ways—had more of an effect on him than it did on others.

Freddie recalled his own childhood as "problem-free," at least until he started junior school. He had got on well with his teachers but vaguely remembered being made to see a support teacher for a number of hours each day for the first few years. However, he had absolutely no recollection of what he had studied with her—he believed that it could possibly have been some form of reading and spelling coaching. He also now remembered that he had experienced tremendous difficulty concentrating at school, but this was only after hearing a lecture on concentration difficulties as part of his nursing training.

In connection with this lecture, he had heard someone say that many children with ADHD were accident-prone. He felt that this statement was certainly true of him—he had been treated in the hospital several times for concussion and arm and leg fractures. He had also been treated once for poisoning after dragging a friend off to the bathroom and finding some medicines they had taken "just to try."

Freddie's GP did not appear really to understand the questions being put to him. He said that he had not heard of any medication for concentration difficulties other than something called ephedrine, which students used to take more than 50 years ago when revising for exams. Freddie remarked that this was precisely the kind of thing he needed. But when his GP nearly laughed, Freddie felt embarrassed to inquire further and left without receiving a proper answer—or any proper help.

Comments

Freddie is an example of a young man for whom things have gone relatively well, despite him likely having had severe ADHD in childhood. His candidness and slightly naïve manner are typical, as was his inability to rephrase his questions during the appointment so that his GP understood the purpose of his visit. (It is also possible, of course, that Freddie's GP may have been totally ignorant in this field and insensitive to his patient's needs.)

Freddie will most probably manage to complete his nursing training without medication (central stimulants). However, he would have undoubtedly benefited from being given a name for his difficulties, which he had correctly identified but had been unable to put into an adequate context.

GILL, 30 YEARS

When Gill noticed the high activity level in her second child, Peter, who was 8 months, she remembered how hard she herself had found it to sit still as a child. At school she had been offered extra reading tuition but had not wished to accept this. Gill had left school after Year 11, having truanted for almost the whole of her final term. She felt that she had always had "ants in her pants," and she was already a heavy smoker at 14 years of age. She had tried to quit smoking while pregnant with her first child but had been unsuccessful. The doctor at the child health center had told her that Peter had bronchitis and was allergic to cigarette smoke and that she now *had to* stop smoking. Gill had no idea how she would manage this and felt just as hounded as she had done during her teens.

Peter started walking at eight months and would rush around the flat, bumping into table edges and pulling things off shelves. He was forever falling over and hurting himself. Gill felt under pressure and grew increasingly impatient. She felt so on edge that she went to see her GP for some tranquilizers. However, her GP did not feel that he could prescribe anything on these grounds and instead offered to refer her to a psychologist for counselling. Gill, though, felt that her situation did not warrant this: she and her husband had a good relationship, she loved her children, and she had no unresolved issues—she simply felt "edgy." Nevertheless her GP insisted, which resulted in Gill seeing a psychologist on three occasions. She did not go back subsequently as she was of the opinion that, if anyone needed help, it was the psychologist, who had not even been able to look her in the eye.

However, a few weeks later, Gill telephoned a private practitioner psychiatrist to request a fairly urgent appointment. She came away from the ensuing consultation with a prescription for 10 non-addictive sleeping tablets. Gill took one and slept until 8 a.m. the following day, resulting in the whole family oversleeping. She then had a headache for the rest of the morning before deciding to return the nine remaining tablets to the chemist.

A month or so later a doctor's appointment for Peter at the child health center arrived in the post. Gill rang the health center nurse and asked whether it would be possible to turn up a few minutes early on the day of the appointment so that she could speak with her. In fact, she was able to see the nurse right away, so she took Peter and went. Gill struck up an instant rapport with her and they talked for over three hours. The nurse confirmed that Peter was more active than was normal and that there could be a connection between Gill's own high activity level and her son's. She added, however, that Peter was still too young for doctors to say whether or not he had a specific diagnosis.

Even though Peter remained a handful, Gill felt calmer following her conversation with the nurse. She also telephoned her mother and chatted with her for longer and in greater depth than she had done in ages. Gill discovered that she had actually been extremely active as a child. Her mother had found this hard work but felt that, if anything, Gill's father had been even more hyper.

Gill realized that Peter's hyperactivity and concentration difficulties were something that ran in the family, and resolved to contend with all of this herself. Her edginess did not subsequently disappear, although the acute sense of chaos and mental breakdown did not recur.

Comments

Gill's story represents a very common problem: a parent who herself has ADHD but who has never received a diagnosis.

Peter will most probably go on to have sufficiently pronounced problems that he will be diagnosed with DAMP or ADHD—but only after several years have elapsed, because neither diagnosis can be made with certainty in a 1-year-old child. If and when Peter is diagnosed, it is very possible that Gill will enquire about herself. Maybe then, at the age of 35, will she learn for the first time that she too has ADHD.

In the future, increasing numbers of adults with these types of difficulties will visit doctors to find out whether they have ADHD/DAMP or another disorder in the ESSENCE group. Knowledge of ADHD/DAMP is growing rapidly in society just as it did in the case of ASD, which was a relatively unknown concept 20 years ago but is now "in general parlance."

Nowadays much is written and spoken about these disorders, and today many adults consult child neuropsychiatrists or adult psychiatrists to discover whether they have, for example, Asperger syndrome. A similar development is likely within the field of ADHD/DAMP. One of the major challenges in the years ahead will be ascertaining how large is the group of adults with childhood-onset ADHD/DAMP who should have access to medication for attention problems and hyperactivity.

HANNAH, 58 YEARS

Hannah's 2-year-old granddaughter was showing signs of strange behaviors such as endlessly walking up and down the same path and insisting that nobody interrupt her, and Hannah knew that everybody was thinking about it although nobody would air their concerns at family meetings or during telephone conversations. Her daughter-in-law had raised the issue of ADHD once; she was a preschool teacher and the children in the nursery where she worked had often been discussed in terms of "hyperactive" and "parenting problems." She was clearly worried, but there was no way that Hannah could voice her own suspicion, lest the fragile truce that she had managed after months of silent fighting with her son would be over in no time.

Hannah, who was still working as a lawyer, was also getting worried about herself, and her memory, thinking, almost on a daily basis, that there must be something bad going on in her head. "Could this be the beginning of Alzheimer's?" "I must remember to remind myself...what was that I was supposed to remember?" "How on earth did I end up here, and what am I doing here?" She was spending much of her time looking for things that she had mislaid (she would say most of the time, but that was not quite true). This was particularly problematic at home, whereas at the workplace, at the law firm, seeing clients, almost on a conveyor belt schedule, she still felt almost "in control."

She had spoken about her concerns regarding possible memory loss to her physician, and he had referred her to an adult psychiatrist who was running a memory clinic. She went there for three visits and was tested twice (for several hours each time) by a neuropsychologist. She complained about her having to remind herself all the time that she needed to do this and that; she would write long lists and then forget where she had put them—once she had found a list in the fridge, and that got her really scared. She told the psychiatrist and the psychologist that she had started writing reminders to herself on her hands and on her lower arms, and she also mentioned to them that one of her clients had pointed this out to her, saying that he would no longer ask for her legal advice seeing as she was in no shape to deal even with her own problems without having to write everything down on her arms.

The neuropsychiatric appraisal came out "normal," and she tested in the superior range on just about everything, except "working memory" and "processing speed." No sign of Alzheimer's, maybe a little depressed mood, maybe she would need to take a break from work, maybe a mild antidepressant? She said she did not feel depressed, but anxious and concerned about her lack of ability to concentrate and to remember what it was that she needed to remember. She looked up "working memory" and "processing speed" on the Internet when she came back from the last visit (she was not going to be followed up, no need for that, she was "fine," except maybe "overworked," it did not matter that she told the psychiatrist that she was actually doing much better at work than at home).

Reading about working memory, she got on to sites mentioning executive dysfunction and then ADHD. She continued to sites describing "female ADHD," and she started thinking: "This is it, this is me, this is what I've got. I have had ADHD all my life, only now is it getting to be such a problem for me that I almost cannot cope." She phoned the psychiatrist's office and asked to have one more consultation.

In preparation for the visit to the psychiatrist, Hannah prepared a short summary of her own background and development. This is what she brought with her to the consultation two weeks later:

I am a 58-year-old woman, successful in work, lawyer (employed) in a law firm, mother of three children, two grandchildren, of whom one female at the age of 2 years is showing some symptoms of ADHD (and possibly also "autistic features"), divorced from father of the children (medical doctor, internist) at 51 years. My parents (according to my mother who is 77 now) had been diagnosed by psychiatrists as suffering from "generalized anxiety disorder" (mother, librarian, but only worked outside of home after the age of 55, often on some kind of psychiatric medication, currently on "SRE" or something?) and "chronic alcoholism" (father, medical doctor, anesthesiologist, died at 64). I have two brothers and a sister, all with some anxiety or drug-related problems. My own eldest son (now 37 years old), the father of my only grandchild, had late onset of speech, spelling problems at school and was always "in trouble," arguing with teachers, poor grades initially, but gradually, with the help of a very understanding class teacher in senior high school, got his "act together." He tested in the above average range on IQ test at age 10 years (school psychologist), but did not go to university, and has worked as a car mechanic since he was 22 after "touring the world" for three years after leaving school. He has been a heavy smoker but quit when his wife got pregnant three years ago. He is a good father, but he has not got along well with me or his father after he came back from the tour around the world. Drug use?

When I was eight I was brought by my parents to a child guidance clinic because I stubbornly refused to eat other than a very few favourite dishes and my school teacher said I was "impossible to keep in a normal classroom" (even though, as far as I can remember, I always attended "normal classes"). I remember having enormous difficulties staying still both in and out of classrooms and being told time and time again to "be quiet." However, I did well (or very well) in most school subjects, but only because I had very "firm" teachers, in subjects where I had lenient teachers I usually only got pass grades or even fail. I was quite young when I had my first son (20), but not as young as my own mother who was only 18 when she had me. My university studies went well and—looking back—I cannot understand how I managed with three children, a husband (who did not help much, according to me), myself, my whole family, studies, work, but somehow the whole thing of having no other choice than to do this, do that, next this, next that, seemed to work wonders for me, and I did well for many years. I remember feeling anxious most of the time though, having difficulty falling asleep at night, but, funnily enough, I regarded myself as quite happy and successful.

Come to think of it, and maybe it is only after reading about ADHD in women on the net that it crossed my mind, but I have always felt as though I am driven by a motor, never being able to wind down, being "high-strung," and I now know (after having asked around a bit during the past week) that that is how other people see me. Well they also say that I am spontaneous and outspoken and that they like me for that but that there is always this "buzz" surrounding me and "things start happening" as soon as I walk in the room.

Comments

Hannah very likely has ADHD and has, of course, had it all her life. Her background and story are typical of females with ADHD, who were not recognized when they were children (and could not have been because the clinical concept of ADHD was not around all those many years ago), and who, during their fertile years and after bearing children, had fewer obvious symptoms of the disorder. In menopause, with the disappearance of estrogen effects on the dopamine system, many of the childhood problems resurface and may even be symptomatically more impairing in many ways than they have ever been before.

The fact that Hannah functions better at work than at home might to some seem surprising. However, the automatic availability in the workplace of "external executive functions," including the structure of seeing clients, one after another, provides a much better ADHD-supporting environment than the unstructured home and leisure time setting of Hannah's out-of-office hours.

The problem she faces now, given her own dawning insight into her basic difficulties, is to convince the psychiatrist that she actually does not have anxiety disorder or depression, but that all her symptoms fit much better with a diagnosis of ADHD. Many adult psychiatrists are almost completely unaware of the clinical presentation of adult ADHD, even though they will have heard about the disorder as it presents in childhood. Will she get a correct diagnosis? Will she be offered better medication for her problems of inattention (which she herself put down to memory failure only a few months ago)?

In the best of worlds, it should be obvious that she would be better off with an ADHD diagnosis than one of mild depression or generalized anxiety disorder, and that a medication trial (with a stimulant or atomoxetine) would probably be appropriate—depending on Hannah's own attitude to such medications. She might be helped a little bit by increasing her intake of omega-3fatty acids, and she would possibly enjoy and make good use of joining a martial arts class or yoga group. Most of all, she would benefit in all sorts of ways from learning more about ADHD and how her own problems fit in with the clinical picture of that diagnosis.

There is no good evidence yet that estrogen therapy could be helpful in a situation like this. However, the theoretical possibility that estrogen would lead to improved dopamine functioning and hence reduced ADHD symptomatology is something that should perhaps be subjected to separate clinical trials, and it is already something that Hannah is considering raising as she prepares for the "extra" meeting with the psychiatrist. She also wishes to discuss the possibility that her grandchild (and maybe her son) might have ADHD, but she wonders whether an adult specialist would be the right person to raise this issue with.